For Anth
with ve
wishes (& thanks
for your heroic
help in the
unwritten sequel!)

love

Peter

November '94

A MIRACLE OF HEALING

Peter Greenhalgh

with illustrations by
Stanley Warburton
and a foreword by

Claire Rayner

MINERVA PRESS
MONTREUX LONDON WASHINGTON

A MIRACLE OF HEALING

ISBN 1 85863 195 5

First Published 1994 by
MINERVA PRESS
2, Old Brompton Road,
London SW7 3DQ.

Printed in Great Britain by
Martins the Printers Ltd., Berwick upon Tweed

A MIRACLE OF HEALING

ABOUT CLAIRE RAYNER

As Britain's favourite "agony aunt", a regular contributor to radio, press and television and author of over 90 books, some of them translated into as many as twelve languages, Claire Rayner is too well known to need much introduction, but not everyone may realise that she began her own career in nursing.

Born in London in 1931, she trained as a nurse at the Royal Northern Hospital, London, where she was awarded the Gold Medal for Outstanding Achievement. After qualifying and becoming State Registered in 1954, she went on to study midwifery at Guy's and later worked at the Royal Free Hospital and the Whittington, where she was a Sister in the Paediatric Department. She married in 1957 and began writing in 1960, when the birth of her first child ended her nursing career.

The knowledge and experience she gained as a nurse are revealed not only in her broad range of writing on medical subjects but also in her novels, as in the fourth volume of her famous Poppy Chronicles where she gives a wonderful evocation of the work of the London Hospital, Whitechapel, in the Blitz. It is therefore particularly appropriate that she kindly offered to write a foreword for a book about that great hospital's work in the 1990's. The author is most grateful to her and touched by the kind words she has written.

ABOUT THE ILLUSTRATOR

Stanley Warburton, born in Lancashire in 1919, is a distinguished water-colourist with work in many public and private collections. He is Vice President of the Turner Society and has advised HRH Prince Charles on his painting.

The author gratefully acknowledges his friend's generosity in doing and donating the evocative pen-and-ink drawings which add so much to this book, royalties from which will go to neurosurgical and rehabilitation charities.

ABOUT THE AUTHOR

Peter Greenhalgh, born in Lancashire in 1945, has shown the versatility of an old-fashioned classical education by dividing his career between the Groves of Academe and the Tempes of Mammon. He has taught Classics and Ancient History at the Universities of Cambridge and Cape Town and been a director of several banks. He currently runs his own international consulting business and is a director of several British and international companies.

His published work includes *Early Greek Warfare* (1973), *The Year of the Four Emperors* (1975), *Pompey: the Roman Alexander* (1980), *Pompey: the Republican Prince* (1981) and *Deep into Mani: A Journey to the southern tip of Greece* (1985, German edition 1987). He has also written and lectured extensively on history, business and corporate finance and is the author of several radio plays, one of which, *The Wrath of Achilles*, won the South African Academy Award for English Radio Drama for 1985.

FOREWORD
by Claire Rayner

I'm going to reveal a trade secret, even at the risk of offending colleagues. In the secret editorial fastnesses of women's magazines, where the articles and stories that will enthral the nation's women are sought for with desperate hunger, there is one kind of piece which everyone knows will work. They're called, with some cynicism in the trade, 'TOTS'. Triumph over tragedy, in other words.

I tell you this so that you will understand what this book is *not*. I suppose there is in the pages a sense of triumph over what might have been a tragedy, but that isn't why I'm so happy to recommend this volume. I do so because it's so much more than that. First of all - and I believe it *does* come first - this is a well written tale that will grab you by the ears and not let you go till the last page. The writing will carry you along so that you're panting to know what happens next. And as a writer whose first rule is, "Thou shalt not be boring," I rate this highly.

Secondly, its fascination is greatly increased by the knowledge that you are being made privy to a true story. I suspect that from the moment we are born we are aching to get inside other people's skins, to see through other eyes, to feel as they do. When you read this story you'll be able to do precisely that. You'll be part of the Greenhalgh family and all they experienced through some of the toughest and most high-keyed months of their lives.

Thirdly, this is an account of something very special about medicine. Yes, the use of high technology in brilliantly fitted units is of prime importance. Yes, the skills of carefully trained doctors, nurses, physios and all the others is of immense value. But here is something else; a sort of human fellow feeling or a power of the mind, or a kind of faith. I don't know what the label is and frankly I don't think it matters. It's enough it exists. The sheer will shared by a lot of people caring for one other person and wanting her to be well.

Clare Greenhalgh had that sort of care at the Trauma Unit of the Royal London Hospital in Whitechapel after a severe head injury. She is today a happy successful young woman - well, almost woman - because of the care she had. Her parents and the people who cared for her are, I think, stronger and better people for what happened. And I suspect that you too, as a reader, will be a wiser person when you've joined them in their experience by reading these pages.

Oh, and just as a bonus - the royalties from the book go to fund this sort of care in the future for other young people who may need it at the Royal London. Doesn't *that* give you a lovely warm fuzzy feeling?

AUTHOR'S PREFACE

This is the true story of a modern miracle of healing. On 4th April, 1992, my daughter had an accident resulting in such serious brain-damage that part of the front left lobe had to be removed in order to save her life. On 10th September, only six months later, she was back at school, mentally and physically unimpaired. I have written her story as a tribute to the modern miracle-workers at Royal London Hospital, Whitechapel, to the police, whose swift action gave her the best chance of recovery, and to the many loved ones and friends, some unknown to us, who supported this work of healing with their love and thoughts and prayers.

At the same time I hope this story may help other parents of children who have to face brain-surgery. Of course, my daughter was one of the very lucky ones. Not all such operations are similarly successful, nor all recoveries so rapid or so complete. But the brain is a remarkably resilient organ, particularly in young people, and the chances of a successful outcome are enormously enhanced if the patient has the benefit of early treatment in a specialised Trauma Unit like that of the London, which is one of this country's great teaching hospitals with a quarter of a millennium of tradition behind it.

This still experimental unit is at the centre of an integrated programme of emergency response to accidents involving brain-damage. It begins with the London's HEMS, the helicopter emergency medical service which can provide immediate resuscitation and ventilation at the scene of an accident, or, in Clare's case, with the police, who were on the spot and commandeered a passing St John ambulance to rush her to a nearby hospital. The Trauma Unit itself is staffed by nurses of the highest technical and professional competence combined with a degree of dedication and humanity that is beyond praise. It is they who support the work of the London's brilliant neurosurgical team in the most critical days, then they in turn hand over to the normal wards and the specialist physiotherapists whose rehabilitation programmes can have the most astonishing results.

To put the success of the integrated Trauma Unit in perspective, the usual expectation in any series of patients of the type which it treats would be for 15 per cent to be left in what is chillingly termed a "persistent vegetative state" (i.e. unable to perform any of the routine daily tasks that we take for granted), and for a further 15 per cent to 20 per cent to be left with such serious disabilities that they cannot live independent lives. To date there have been no such outcomes at all since the Unit opened. The savings in terms of human suffering - not to mention the savings in the financial cost of maintaining highly dependent patients for life - are incalculable, and I hope this little book will result in a wider knowledge and appreciation of these remarkable achievements, particularly at a time when the whole future of London's great teaching hospitals is under debate. Great hospitals are like great regiments: an *esprit de corps* that has taken centuries to create can be destroyed overnight by the stroke of a bureaucrat's pen.

The experience my wife and I have been through has given us a better perspective on life and what is important in it. It has also restored our faith in human nature, the bad side of which seems to dominate the interest of so many of the media nowadays. We were shown so much kindness by so many people. The much-maligned police, for example, not only rescued Clare and traced us with great efficiency but rang the hospital regularly for several days to enquire how she was until she was out of danger. The staff of the hospital - surgeons, anaesthetists, nurses, physiotherapists, the Chaplaincy and all the ancillary staff - were without exception very caring people: theirs was more than just a job of work to be done, and how they stand the emotional as well as the physical and mental strains I simply do not know. Then there were our friends, relatives and neighbours, our church and the congregations of friends' churches in many parts of the world who prayed for Clare without even knowing her. For there is nothing mutually exclusive in healing by prayer and by the skills of modern medical science. A healing is no less a miracle because the hands 'laid on' have scalpels or syringes in them.

Few things seem to me more naive and offensive than the mass faith-healing sessions held in sports stadiums by tele-evangelists who insult the sick and crippled by accusing them of lack of faith. Nor is there anything sadder or blinder than the scientist who cannot see the workings of divine intelligence in his achievements but somehow attributes the development of his infinitely complex mental and physical faculties to a series of evolutionary 'accidents' devoid of design. My own eyes have certainly been opened, and I have both felt and observed the efficacy of prayer in support of all the God-given skills of the modern miracle-workers, whether or not they recognise it themselves. If it is true that God helps those who help themselves, it is even truer that He helps those who help others, and that it is more blessed to give than to receive. We have been given the supreme blessing of having our daughter restored to us in a condition of health beyond all expectation. But what is our blessing to that of those who gave it to us and whose story is told with a father's deepest gratitude in this book?

This book is gratefully dedicated to the Royal London Hospital's Trauma Unit, its surgical, medical, nursing, physiotherapy, chaplaincy and support staff, its Helicopter Emergency Medical Service, the Metropolitan Police, St. John Ambulance and all who contribute to modern miracles of healing everywhere.

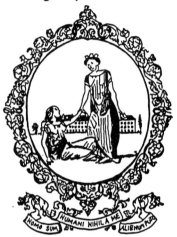

This drawing is of the seal made for the London Hospital in 1758 by John Ellicott, a member of its Court of Governors. The Ellicotts were a wealthy and philanthropic family of watchmakers, and among their gifts to the hospital was the great clock over the main entrance in Whitechapel Road.

The crowned 'Lady Samaritan' reaching down to help the injured young woman to rise is Londinia, the tutelar goddess of London whose castellated crown represents the city wall. The building in the background is the hospital itself, then of course new and in a still semi-rural setting before the Industrial Revolution transformed the East End into a pre-Blitz version of what we see today. This female variation of the Good Samaritan theme depicted by Hogarth in his great painting at St. Bart's is a particularly appropriate design for a book about the modern healing of a young woman by the Royal London.

The Latin motto, taken from Terence's play *Heautontimorumenos,* is a good one for a caring profession in a selfish age. "I am a human being: I consider no human concern to be a matter of indifference to me."

CHAPTER ONE

It is the moment every parent dreads - the knock on the door by the police. 'Your daughter has had an accident - it's serious I'm afraid. You must come to the hospital at 'once'.

The beginning of this nightmare for us was 8.30 p.m. on Saturday, 4th April, 1992. Our daughter, Clare, was then fourteen, a bright and cheerful girl, tall for her age and looking seventeen - a mixed blessing - but not too badly spoilt for an only child. On the fateful Saturday morning she had been rung up by a school friend, a Yugoslav girl called Marta who had spent a term in Clare's class while her father had been working in London. The school had just broken up for the Easter holidays, and Marta's father was about to go to work in Switzerland and take her with him. In fact they were off the next day, and Marta had rung to see if Clare could come and spend the last afternoon with her.

Unfortunately Marta lived much too far away to make this possible, but the ever-resourceful Clare rang two of her other friends and asked if they would join her in an expedition to London to meet Marta there and buy her a farewell present. As they were both keen to do so and their parents agreed, we could not really refuse the *fait accompli* with which Clare presented us. But there were conditions. Mary, my wife, would drive Clare in to Charing Cross station and see that she met up with Marta and her two other friends, all of whom were coming in by train. That rendezvous was fixed for 3.30, then the girls could go together to Covent Garden, only a short walk away, with the promise to stick together and return to the station about half past five. Clare was then to ring home and we could meet her off the train at one of the two local stations, Blackheath or Lewisham.

It seemed safe enough. Clare is a responsible girl, and she was particularly on 'best behaviour' as she was due to go to Italy in a few days' time with a school party from her Italian class for the first leg of an exchange visit with girls in Montepulciano, a town in Tuscany which sounded delightful. Besides, the other girls were all a year older, and if they stuck together they could surely come to little harm visiting Covent Garden to buy a friend a farewell present on a Saturday afternoon. But 5.30 came and went, then 6 o'clock, then 6.30, and still no call from Clare. At this stage we were more annoyed than worried. If she had wanted to stay a bit longer, surely she could have rung. She usually did, to stop the old 'fuss-pots' from fussing, and certainly this fuss-pot was preparing some serious words for his thoughtless daughter on her return. But when 7 o'clock came and there was still no news, we began to feel uneasy. We rang the parents of Clare's companions. The phone of one was out of order and there was no reply from the second, but we got through to Alice's mother and were reassured to hear that she had not returned either. As long as they were together they should be all right, but really it was too bad of Clare, especially as she had promised faithfully to ring...

Even though the clocks had recently been put forward for Summer time, it was already getting dark, and by 8 o'clock we were becoming quite alarmed. Then at last the telephone rang. But it was not Clare. It was Alice's mother saying that Alice had just returned home in Orpington and told her that Clare had left to come home a full hour before she had. Apparently the other girls had wanted to stay an extra hour, but Clare had said she had promised to be home on time and had left as planned before half past five to walk back to Charing Cross station. It was only a short step from Covent Garden, and though they had promised to keep together, well, it was no distance...

Mary now rang the police and gave a description of Clare. 'A fourteen-year-old, about 5 feet 8 inches tall and looking about seventeen. Wearing a black leather jacket, jeans and a pair of those army-type boots that are all the rage'. It sounded awful. The police asked if she had ever 'absconded' before, had she people she might visit? Even as Mary said, 'No, she is a good girl, she is always careful to ring and be back on time', it sounded hollow. Don't they all say that? Anyway, the police said they would put out a description and let us know.

If Clare had not come back there were only two possibilities. One was an accident, the other could be something even worse. Had she been picked up by someone, got into someone's car despite all the warnings we had given her? Or was it possible, as the police had suggested, that she had absconded? Surely not. But do parents always know their daughters as well as they believe? Was it just possible? All I knew for certain was that I could not just sit and wait for the telephone to ring. I got hold of the first three photographs of Clare I could find, one a school photo and two from a recent holiday in Crete, one of which showed her tucking into a huge concoction of ice cream and fruit salad. My hand was shaking as I put them in my pocket. Then I set out to drive to our two local stations to see if the ticket-collectors or porters had noticed her.

I went first to Lewisham, but the ticket-collector there was lolling against the side of his box talking to a friend and not troubling to look at tickets, let alone the passengers themselves. He could not help and resented having his conversation interrupted. Then I went to Blackheath Station, which is separated from our house by the heath itself. Clare is strictly forbidden to walk on it alone in the dark, but I watched carefully to see if she was walking down the road which crosses it. At the station there was no ticket-collector or porter on duty at all, but a train was just coming in from London. A lot of young people got out, and I watched them anxiously for Clare. Surely she would come. She must. But no - the happy chattering tide of passengers flowed past me and left me alone on the platform. There was nothing to do but go back home and see if Mary had heard anything. If not, I thought I should drive in to Charing Cross and ask there, though the chances of her having been noticed in that enormous station must be minimal. Still, I could at least find out if there had been an accident in the area.

As I walked up the short path to the house I saw a big piece of paper sticking out of the letterbox. It was from Mary. 'She has had an accident. Westminster Hospital, Horseferry Road. The police are taking me, please come now. I love you'. It is impossible to describe my feelings at that moment. I felt stunned, as though I had received a physical blow, and as I looked stupidly at the paper in my hand, disbelief still contended with proof for a moment before I pulled myself together, opened the door and ran in to telephone the hospital, to find out if Clare was alive and exactly where it was.

I had no sooner found the number in the directory than the phone rang and it was Mary. She was controlling herself bravely. Yes, Clare was alive but had had a serious accident and injured her head and chest. She was in Intensive Care, but Mary had not been able to see her yet. Yes, I would come at once. Then as Mary tried to explain where the hospital was, the phone was taken from her by one of the staff who gave me clear directions, and I set off at once.

My own journey was evidently less rapid than Mary's, though I went pretty fast. Shooting across one junction I got an outraged blast

on the horn from another driver, and thought how often I had done the
same to someone else without ever thinking that there might be a
better reason for the other chap's haste than macho aggression or plain
idiocy. Near Westminster Bridge I went twice round the one-way
system because I had forgotten my glasses and being short-sighted I
had not been able to read the signs until it was too late. All the same
I covered fifteen very built-up miles in twenty-five minutes. The
police, however, had done it in half that time, so Mary told me later.
'Get in the back, love, and put the seat belt on', they had said. 'We'll
be moving'. And move they certainly did, touching an incredible 100
miles per hour down the Old Kent Road.

Mary had not known if Clare was *alive* or not until she reached the
hospital. All the police had been able to tell her was that it was very
serious as it was their highest category of emergency and one rarely
used. At least I had known that she was alive when I was driving in.
The entrance to the Westminster Hospital is in a side street, and I
remember walking in past an ambulance, another police car and a sad
little knot of down-and-out young people presumably waiting for some
friend who had been admitted. But I had no sooner inquired for Clare
at the desk than Mary appeared on the stairs and we went up together
to Intensive Care.

It was only later that I was able to piece together what had
happened. About 5.30 the girls were enjoying themselves so much
wandering around the shops and boutiques of Covent Garden that the
other three had decided to stay another hour but Clare, following
instructions for once, said she would have to get back. Yes, of course
she would be all right. It was only a short walk down to the Strand,
then straight along to Charing Cross Station. When she reached the
Strand, however, she saw a bus coming along, jumped on, then
jumped off again outside the station. Unfortunately it was one of the
old-style buses without doors and she did what we have all done
scores of times, jumping off just before it had completely stopped.
The trick of course is to run forward as you touch the ground and
keep the momentum going, but Clare somehow overbalanced and fell
heavily onto the kerb, fracturing her skull and breaking some ribs.

Mercifully there was a van-load of policemen just behind the bus
on their way to a political demonstration in Trafalgar Square. They
saw it all, piled out and gave her first aid. At first she spoke to them,
and though her head was bleeding they thought she was just badly

concussed; but then she was very sick, lost consciousness and began to go cold. Realising that it was something very serious, they were just about to radio for an ambulance when they spotted an empty St John's one which happened to be passing, also on its way to the Trafalgar Square demonstration. They commandeered it at once, then leading the way with sirens wailing they rushed Clare into the nearest hospital, the Westminster, and set about tracing her parents.

All children - and all grown-ups for that matter - should carry a note of their name, address, telephone number and numbers to contact in an emergency. We know better now, but the only means of identification which Clare had with her that day was her Woolwich Building Society account card, which gave only her name and account number. The police, however, got in touch with the Branch Manager at his home, and he rushed to the office to find her address. In the meantime the Greenwich police to whom we had reported that Clare was missing had circulated her name and description, but it was just after the Westminster police had discovered her address that the two were connected. Anyway, Clare was safely in hospital by that time, and we were now with her.

The Intensive Care Unit was on the second floor. I remember the double doors leading across a long corridor which led to other wards to the right and to the radiology department to the left. The Intensive Care Unit itself was straight across, with a kind of vestibule which had a storeroom on the right and a tiny administrative office on the left with a desk, a couple of chairs and a small library. It was here that Mary had been put when she arrived, but she had still not seen Clare as the doctors were desperately trying to restore her body-temperature, which had fallen dangerously low. She was having blood-transfusions and was on the full life-support systems, her breathing controlled by a ventilator. One of the doctors came to us briefly to explain what was happening and said that it would be a little time yet before we were able to go to Clare. In the meantime we were brought cups of strong sweet tea, the first of many. Dear old stand-by. It is somehow such a homely and comforting drink, and the kindness with which it was brought was much appreciated.

It was about twenty minutes before we were able to go in and see Clare, and when we did it was fairly grim. Her hair was matted with blood, her eyes black and terribly swollen, her whole face elongated by heavy swelling round the neck and jaws. She was, of course, unconscious, her life depending on the bewildering battery of machines to which she was connected. And she was so cold. As I stroked her poor limbs a shudder went through me as I remembered where I had felt skin like that before: it was when I had held my dead father's hand for a moment in the Chapel of Rest the day before his funeral. It is hard to express what Mary and I now felt as we looked helplessly at our pretty fourteen-year-old daughter, our only child, in such a terrible mess. If only I could have changed places with her. 'If only'. How many times we would use that useless expression that night and in the days that followed.

The senior doctor kindly took us back to the little room and said that he was going to try to get her into another hospital. He could not say how serious the damage was, but he would feel happier if she was in a hospital with a specialist neurosurgical unit. In the meantime their top priority was to get her body-temperature up and he said she seemed at last to be responding to the transfusions. He also said he was frankly puzzled at the amount of damage that seemed to have been done by a low-velocity injury, not only to the head but also to her chest. But when I said this to a scientist friend of mine a few days later, he pointed out that her head was not exactly travelling at a low velocity if it hit the pavement from vertical purely from the force of gravity, let alone from the jolt she would have received. The speed of impact when I worked it out would have been about 45 miles per hour. Just imagine a child's head being hit by a car going at that speed.

By now it must have been about 10.30 at least, and though I knew he went to bed early (because he is early to rise) I rang a very dear friend who is Professor of Neurovirology at St Thomas's, Hughie Webb. Poor Hughie was indeed in bed and asleep, but doctors are used to being awakened by someone else's nightmares, and he was typically kind without wrapping anything up. From my answers to his questions he told me it was evidently very serious but he reassured me that the Westminster staff were doing all the right things and were also wise to seek to transfer her to a specialist neurosurgical department. He said that the National at Queen's Square was one of the best specialist hospitals for brain damage and disease, but there were other good ones too. I should let him know as soon as possible what had been arranged. In the meantime there was no point in saying 'Don't worry' but the brain, he said, had great powers of recovery from even the most terrible accidents, and Clare had youth on her side.

When I returned from making my phone call I met the doctor again at the door to our little room. He had come to tell us that he had secured a bed for Clare at the National, and we felt very relieved. But before moving her they wanted to try and get her body-temperature a bit higher, and in the meantime, as their consultant radiologist had just come in on another matter, he would give her a brain scan. About ten minutes later we watched Clare's bed, festooned with all its paraphernalia, being wheeled away down the dimly lit corridor to the X-ray department. We felt so utterly helpless and useless. There was nothing even to say. We simply held hands and went back to sit and wait as patiently as we could in the little office. I noticed a book in the bookcase on the nursing of brain-damaged patients, but it was so horrific that I soon put it back. And during the next half hour or so while we waited for news I took in all the details of that room, which are now so many pieces of useless knowledge cluttering up my own decaying memory cells.

It is odd how trivial things become imprinted on one's mind at times of crisis. Most of all I am afraid I remember the filthy state of the desk-top computer. It was clearly in use because some keys were relatively clean from the pressure of fingers, but the rest of them, and the spaces between them, were caked with grime, the screen itself was filthy, the whole thing frankly disgusting. However good the medical and nursing care, that computer was a disgrace to the administration and cleaners. I could not imagine how anyone could bear to use the thing in that condition, and while I have nothing but praise and gratitude for the excellent care which Clare received, I could not help feeling that there was a lot wrong with the administration of that hospital. In the corridor outside, for example, cupboard doors were all half open, boxes of medical supplies had been thrown into higgledy-piggledy heaps on the shelves, and I was astonished to see one very senior person - who in the old days would have been called Matron but now had a badge with some grandiose administrative title several words long - walk down that corridor several times either without noticing or without caring about the shambolic state of the cupboards, or bits of tubing lying on the floor (to be kicked out of the way rather than picked up), or a filthy old slipper that was lying right in the entrance to the ward.

When Clare returned from the CT scan about an hour later, the radiologist came to see us. He was a cheerful soul, an Ulsterman to judge by his accent, and he said that although the pictures had not been as clear as he would have liked he felt there was a reasonable chance that the brain damage would not prove too severe, though there was internal bleeding causing pressure in the skull and this was the most critical aspect. He too said that he was surprised that so much damage had been done. He said he was always doing 'head-snaps' of foreign tourists who were constantly getting hit by cars in Westminster as they looked the wrong way crossing the road, and he had become rather blasé about it. But Clare had evidently done far more damage to her head than would have been expected from a simple fall, and he fully agreed with his colleague that she should be transferred to a specialist neurosurgical hospital without delay.

About midnight the doctor who had told us that he had secured a bed for Clare in the National now came in to say that he was sending her to the London Hospital in Whitechapel instead. While the National was ideal for brain damage, he explained, they could not deal with thoracic problems, and he was worried about Clare's chest as well as her head. He was afraid that the fractured ribs might have done some internal damage too, for though, mercifully, they had not punctured a lung, there was serious bruising in there and it would be wiser for her to be in a hospital with specialist departments in both areas.

The mention of Whitechapel struck me with a dull thud. I knew it only as a very rough area of decaying tenements housing sweat-shops where the former Jewish workers have been largely replaced by Bangladeshis making cheap clothing for a pittance, and everything that has fallen off the back of a truck is for sale on stalls in streets where you don't park your car if you want to see its wheels again. Yes, such is its reputation, and though exaggerated it is not entirely unjustified. But every coin has two sides, and the reverse side is much brighter and rings truer. As Clare was being prepared for the transfer, I rang Hughie Webb again and told him where she was going. His reply was unequivocal. 'The London has a superb neurosurgical department, and if Clare has thoracic problems too, they could not do better'. How right he was is something which we were to prove for ourselves and which is why this book has been written, for the London Hospital in darkest Whitechapel - or rather the 'Royal

London' as it has been since 1990 when the Queen gave it that title to celebrate its 250th anniversary - could not, I believe, be bettered anywhere in the world.

CHAPTER TWO

At that time of night there was nothing on the road and the journey to Whitechapel was a fast one even for me, following the ambulance at first but inevitably losing it at the first red light. Mary travelled with Clare in the ambulance together with a doctor and nurse who attended to her ventilation, transfusion and all the portable drips and monitors which went with her. I parked outside the front of the London Hospital, and as I was walking through the main entrance I met Clare being trundled through from the Admission area to the lifts which led up to Intensive Care, or rather the Intensive Therapy Unit (ITU) as they now call it. I suppose 'therapy' is a better word than 'care' because it sounds more positive, indicating active treatment and improvement. It is on the third floor, which also has the operating suites. Clare disappeared inside, and after a quarter of an hour or so the doctor and nurse from the Westminster came out, having handed her over to the staff of the London, and we said a very appreciative good-bye. They were genuinely concerned people - it was more than just professional competence - and throughout our experience of the weeks ahead we were constantly heartened and humbled to find among the clinical and nursing staff a combination of professionalism and humanity that was quite beyond praise.

A nurse came out a little later and showed us to a small sitting room kept especially for the relatives of patients in ITU. It was furnished with some easy chairs, some tea-making equipment and a small fridge, and there was an adjoining bathroom-cum-kitchen with a sink and a shower. We found an elderly Irish couple there whose brother was in ITU and very seriously ill. They showed us where the mugs and tea were kept and kindly made us a cup. By one of those extraordinary coincidences it turned out that they too lived in Blackheath, not more than a few hundred yards from us. There is a natural camaraderie among people in distress, and as we sat together waiting it gave us a sense of what it must have been like in the War.

After about half an hour a nurse came to fetch us and we saw Clare briefly, looking very much the same as she had done in the Westminster. We were told that the Senior Registrar in Neurosurgery had seen her and decided that it was necessary to implant a brain-pressure monitor in her head. They were preparing her for theatre right away as this required a minor operation to drill a hole in the skull to insert a metal sensor. A younger member of the neurosurgical team, Dr John Britto, asked me to sign the consent form. He reassured us that it was a routine procedure involving no risk but they were worried about the pressure building up in the skull, and it was literally vital to monitor this. 'The brain is a wonderfully resilient organ', he explained, 'but it has the disadvantage of being confined in a very tight box. If it is bruised and starts to swell, serious and permanent damage can be done'.

After I had signed the form we watched as Clare's bed, with a cluster of attendants looking after all the machinery which went with her, was wheeled out of ITU, past the little relatives' room and through the double doors which led to the corridor of operating theatres. We saw her disappear into theatre no. 8, then took up our station on two stacking chairs that happened to be sitting at the top of the stairwell. One was blue, the other red, and they got to know our bottoms quite well over the next twenty-four hours. Somehow we did not feel like going back into the relatives' room to wait. We wanted to be by ourselves and, I suppose, as near as possible to Clare.

The minutes passed so slowly. Through the glass panel in the double doors we caught glimpses of gowned figures moving up and down the dimly lit corridor with sudden bursts of bright light as they went in or out of the operating theatres on either side, but it was over an hour before Clare emerged, and when she did she was taken not to ITU but to the specialist Trauma Unit. This was a ward of only four beds with two, or sometimes three, very highly trained nursing staff to attend to them. Whereas ITU itself deals with the intensive care of both surgical and medical patients, the Trauma Unit is limited mainly to neurosurgical cases resulting from serious accidents and usually involving brain damage. To some extent the Unit is still experimental because arguments seem to rage in medical circles about the need for such a high degree of specialisation. All I can say, after seeing what the Trauma Unit did for Clare and others in the many hours we were to spend there, is that it is something which needs cloning and developing in similar centres of excellence all over the country. The danger is that innovation always has its detractors, and if insufficient resources are put behind a new unit or it is rather grudgingly given inadequate premises and staffing 'to see how it goes', it is not being given a fair chance and is more likely to confirm what become self-fulfilling prophecies of failure. Just because the atom was smashed in little more than an attic, it does not follow that attics are the best places to smash them.

The speed with which accident victims receive expert attention is literally vital in many cases, and even where it does not mean the difference between life and death, it can still mean the difference between a good recovery and permanent disability. Clare was fortunate in having the immediate attention of the police, who commandeered the passing ambulance and had her under the care of the resuscitation team at the Westminster in a matter of minutes. But what would have happened if she had not been so near a major hospital, or had been stuck in traffic without the specialist attention? With luck she would have been collected by the Helicopter Emergency Service, which is based on the London Hospital and is the reason why a specialised Trauma Unit was established separately from the more general Intensive Therapy department.

Helicopters are very much used as ambulances in other countries but we have been slow here to make use of what is clearly the fastest and most versatile form of transport. I suppose it boils down to cost, but in 1988 the *Daily Express* newspaper set up a charity to buy, equip and run a helicopter, and the Department of Health paid for the London's rooftop helipad and its dedicated lift straight down to the emergency admissions room. It is a superbly integrated operation. The helicopter can be at the site of an accident in minutes, and the pilots are so skilled that they have even managed to put down in Oxford Circus. Treatment begins immediately. The helicopter is not just a means of rapid transport but a flying intensive care unit with a doctor, a paramedic and the complete resuscitation kit of ventilators, ECG monitors, defibrillator, pulse oximeter, blood-oxygen monitors, vacuum mattresses, infusors, suction and much of the other equipment with which we were to become so familiar in the Trauma Unit. Trauma specialists refer to the 'Golden Hour' in which aggressive resuscitation and prompt surgical intervention after an accident can reduce the number of early hospital deaths dramatically and save many patients who would otherwise die or be severely impaired through internal haemorrhage in the head, chest or abdomen. In computing the cost-effectiveness of the service there should be vast allowance for the saved expense to the Health Service of patients requiring treatment for life because they did not receive the specialist early intervention which could have avoided permanent damage. As to the non-monetary aspect of saving a young mind, what value can be put on that?

When Clare came out of theatre we had to wait another half hour or so while they settled her into the Trauma Unit, but the lady anaesthetist had a word with us and said we should be able to see her as soon as possible. When we did, it was horrifying, but Mary was wonderfully controlled as we sat beside Clare's bed, holding her hands and praying and willing her to recover. She seemed to have tubes and wires everywhere. The ventilator which breathed for her covered her nose and mouth, there were ECG terminals on her chest, and transfusion points had been inserted in her hands, feet and neck, some with tubes attached, some with little taps on them ready to be opened for injections into the veins or arteries as necessary. And now there was a strange metal spike sticking out of her skull with wires attaching it to two monitors, one of which I gathered was a new type which they wanted the opportunity of testing. Banks of monitor screens above her head showed constantly flickering columns of figures while others plotted eerie green graphs of heart-beat, blood-oxygen and - most critically - the pressure in the brain. Huge charts had been set out on a table at the foot of the bed, and every few minutes readings were taken, graphs plotted and adjustments made to the type and speed of the fluids that were being pumped into Clare. Every so often injections would be given through one of the vein or artery taps on her neck, arm or leg, and all the time the ventilator kept her breathing steadily, effortlessly, to give her battered body and brain the chance to recover.

A physiotherapist came in from time to time and helped to get the fluid off Clare's lungs, which had been badly bruised but mercifully not punctured by the broken ribs. Apparently the broken ribs themselves were of no consequence as they rapidly knit together again of their own accord, particularly in young people. But there was a lot of fluid accumulating in the lungs, and Linda was an expert at getting rid of it. She was very petite, not nearly as tall as Clare, but immensely strong and highly skilled. She would deftly roll Clare onto her side then strike her back hard several times with one hand laid over the other. In the meantime a nurse had inserted a tube down Clare's throat through the ventilator mouthpiece and connected it to a suction machine. The appalling convulsions of coughing that followed

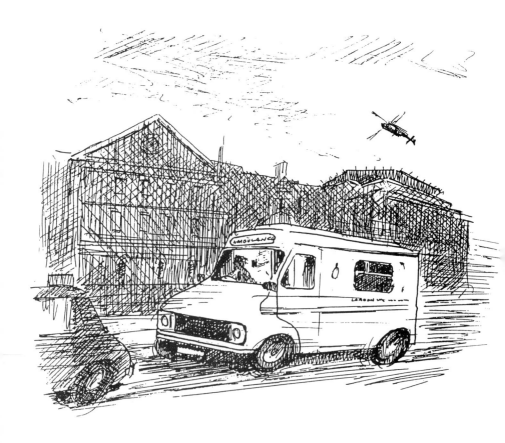

were awful to watch, but it was a case of being cruel to be kind. It was vital to get the fluid up, and soon the suction bottle had an amazing quantity in it, all carefully measured and recorded. But despite the internal upheavals, only Clare's left hand and leg had moved a bit, and there was no flicker of consciousness. Her swollen eyes remained tightly closed and her poor face looked as impassive as a Greek icon, strangely elongated by the swelling of her neck and with great black unseeing eyes, clearly not belonging to this world. The only encouraging sign was that she was now warming up nicely, her limbs no longer having that terrible corpse-like feeling they had had a few hours earlier.

The neurosurgical team came in and explained again that their main concern was the pressure in the brain. The monitors were showing it at well over 20, which was the danger level in whatever units it was being measured. The brain was evidently damaged in two areas, one over the right eye where the skull had been fractured and the other, more worryingly, behind the left front temple, which was coming under increasing pressure as the brain had been thrown hard against that part of the skull by the force of the blow.

They had no way of knowing if there were other areas of bruising deeper within the brain where they could not be detected by the CT scans, but we were warned that surgery might be necessary if the pressure did not come down soon. In the meantime they were administering a drug that actually shrank the brain in the hope of reducing the pressure sufficiently to stabilise the swelling and avoid having to operate.

We naturally became obsessed with watching that monitor now, or rather both of them, and trying to will them to go down. Sometimes the numbers dropped into the teens and our hopes rose, but a few moments later they would be up in the twenties, thirties, forties or even higher. Sometimes they remained in a fairly small band for a short time but at other times they would flicker madly up and down in sudden bursts of activity. The monitors clicked on remorselessly. '22, 22, 21, 20, 20...yes, yes, please keep going down...20, 20, 19, 18, 17, 17, 15...that's better, keep going', but then it would shoot up again just as quickly to 25, 30, 35, 40 or even 60. Doses were adjusted, charts filled in. Calmly, competently and kindly the Trauma nurses went about their exacting work, and Clare was not their only charge. In the second of the four beds was a man equally ill, also on ventilation and linked up, like Clare, to every conceivable support and monitoring system. And in the third bed was an old lady, relatively peaceful and requiring less concentrated attention as she was not being ventilated. One nurse was generally with Clare while her colleague was with the man, but every so often they would join forces to perform a task requiring more than one pair of hands, or to bring something for one another, or to consult. It was a long and exhausting twelve hours for them.

Dawn came at last and with it the helicopter, which roosts overnight at Biggin Hill aerodrome in Kent and comes at dawn to its perch on the roof of the London Hospital. The helipad is visible from the Trauma Unit's windows and we first heard and then saw the helicopter clattering down to land. Then a few moments later we saw the flying doctor himself, a dashing-looking young man wearing an orange flying suit, flying boots and a big luminous sign saying 'DOCTOR' on his back. He had heard that a teenage accident victim had come into the Trauma Unit during the night and wanted to check how she had been admitted and why the helicopter had not been called the previous afternoon. 'We could have brought her straight here from the scene of the accident yesterday if we had only been notified' he said, and he clearly thought that the emergency services had been inefficient. But he relaxed when we explained that no 999 call had been made because the police and a St John's ambulance had been on the spot, and when he heard how quickly Clare had been got into the full resuscitation treatment at the Westminster he thought they had done well.

Clare, who often talked about going into the RAF, would have loved to meet this dashing young flying doctor, and as we stood over the poor soul lying limp, battered and unconscious, I think he must have read my mind because he said, 'Don't worry, I've brought in worse than Clare, and they have made marvellous recoveries'. Then he told me about another fourteen-year-old girl, Vicky, whom he had brought in five weeks ago. 'She had had a terrible accident and had to have some very serious brain surgery to save her life. But she is fine now, or at least she will be as soon as her leg is mended. Her head's OK'. The nurses too had told us about Vicky during the night, and later that day we were to meet her.

At 8 o'clock in the morning the day-staff came on duty, and there was a very careful handover with charts pored over and every detail of each patient's condition and treatment minutely discussed. Nor were the parents forgotten. We had dozed intermittently while sitting with Clare during the night but arrangements were now being discussed for us to be given a room to sleep in. There was one bedroom for relatives just opposite the Trauma Unit itself, but as this was currently occupied by the parents of a child in ITU we were given a room in James Hora House, which is a whole hostel for the accommodation of relatives of critically ill patients and also for patients themselves who have to visit the hospital for regular courses of treatment (radiotherapy or chemotherapy for example) but do not need nursing care. It is a delightful house and very convenient, being just off the main courtyard of the hospital. It has thirteen bedrooms, a kitchen-cum-breakfast room, bathrooms, a laundry room and two lounges, one for smokers and one smoke-free. I am not certain but I think it is a unique facility among major hospitals in the whole country, not just Greater London. A lady Superintendent and her deputy take turns to live in, and as they are both qualified social workers they are able to help with both the practical and the emotional problems of their residents. It is a marvellous facility for a hospital to have, and entirely free of charge. Residents are simply invited to make a donation according to their means when they leave. The main financial support comes from the Marie Celeste Samaritan Society, a charity which celebrated its two-hundredth anniversary in 1991 and has a fascinating history.

In 1791 one of the surgeons at the London, William Blizzard, decided to do something about the lack of any provision for poor patients when they left hospital and the appalling distress that often resulted. He therefore founded what was then called simply 'The Samaritan Society' with the motto 'Take care of him' - the words of the Good Samaritan to the Innkeeper when he left a sum of money to enable the injured man to be cared for - 'and whatsoever thou spendest more, when I come again I will repay thee'. The Society's work expanded rapidly to meet such needs as supplying patients with spectacles, artificial limbs, clothing and trusses. Blizzard was a pioneer of the follow-up care without which so much of the work of healing can be wasted if it ends when the patient leaves the hospital gates. What is taken for granted now was an innovation then, but his detractors were soon silenced by his success, for already in 1795 it was recorded that 'many poor patients in the London Hospital, after they had been cured of their diseases and were in a state of convalescence, had been supplied with necessaries and enabled to return home and renew their occupations'. Then a little over a century later the Society gained a new lease of life and its present name, when in 1898 the wealthy Victorian philanthropist, James Hora, bequeathed a large part of his very large fortune to it in memory of his first wife, Marie Celeste. He had long felt remorse that he had not taken enough care of her when they were living in Australia, where she was very unhappy while he was making money, and to perpetuate her memory he asked for her name to be associated with the hospital. And while her name is perpetuated both in the name of the Society and the Marie Celeste maternity wards which he endowed, his own name is preserved in that of the James Hora hostel in which we were now privileged to stay.

The Superintendent kindly came over to the Trauma Unit and took us over to the hostel herself, then made us a cup of tea and showed us round. As we had nothing with us except the now rather revolting clothes we stood up in, we decided that I should go back home quickly and bring some things. It took me only about twenty-five minutes to drive home as there was little traffic on the roads so relatively early on a Sunday morning, but when I walked into the empty house I was quite unprepared for the feeling of utter desolation that swept over me. I had with me a plastic bag full of Clare's clothes which they had given me at the Westminster - her jeans, boots, T-shirt, pants and the black leather jacket caked with dried blood all down the back. I dumped this quickly in the cellar without daring to open it again, then fed her goldfish and budgerigar in the kitchen and went upstairs to collect some fresh clothes and washing things for Mary and me. Finally I went up to Clare's room on the second floor, as the nurses had suggested that I bring a few of her personal and favourite things - her favourite soap and deodorant for example, a few tapes which she liked listening to, a teddy bear, all things that might create some recognition, even sub-consciously. So far I had managed to keep my emotions under control, but the sight of Clare's gloriously untidy room in which every single thing seemed stamped with her personality was more than I could bear. On the wall was a lovely photograph of Clare with her favourite horse at a little farm in Lancashire where she loves to go and stay. But would she ever walk again, let alone ride Dante? Would she read her books, listen to her records, go back to school? I began sobbing uncontrollably, and throwing myself on my knees by her bed I prayed as I had never prayed before.

Prayer has never been easy for me. I do not mean the liturgical prayer of the Church of England to which I was brought up and whose services I used to love for the beauty of their language before they were modernised to the point where even the Lord's Prayer sometimes breaks down nowadays in Church because the old, well-loved words have been changed. The prayer I find difficult is private prayer, particularly for help in one's own needs. The voice of logic at the back of my mind tells me that my problems are infinitesimal in the scale of things. Why should my prayer be listened to when countless millions are suffering throughout the world from poverty, pestilence, natural disasters (the so-called 'acts of God') or human oppression and cruelty? So generally I pray for the strength to look after my family and to try to do some good in the very limited area which I have some hope of affecting. But now I was confronted with an intensely personal need which no strength of mine or money or any action at all on my part could possibly help, except, paradoxically, by prayer. I was totally dependent on the skill and strength of others to save Clare - the doctors and nurses who had her in their care.

Praying for the general amelioration of suffering in distant lands stricken with war or epidemics or flood or drought is surely right, but even then its best effect must be to actuate the person praying to give money or time or both, to use his own strength and capabilities to give practical assistance. This, after all, is what Christ himself did, encouraging the rich and pious young man to help the poor, giving the example of the Samaritan for practical assistance to the sufferer. And when he healed people himself, it was always on a personal basis, one to one. He never healed suffering populations in distant lands, cured the plague victims of Corinth or diverted the floods of the Indus. His was a personal ministry, and his healings were usually made by physical contact, often actively - by laying his hands on the blind or lame - but sometimes passively, as when the woman with a haemorrhage touched his garment and he felt the strength go out of him. There is, however, one healing at a distance, and I have always thought it the most moving of the miracles and the one least likely to be fictional. It is still strictly personal in the sense that Christ was healing one specific person of whom he had knowledge, but he had never met that person: the healing was done from afar by faith, and this was the sort of faith which I now prayed to have.

It is the wonderful story of the Roman Centurion, which is told in the gospels of both Matthew and Luke. Fearing for the life of a dearly loved member of his household, this high-ranking Roman officer sent and asked Jesus to heal him. Jesus agreed to come, but the Centurion said that this was surely unnecessary, and in any case he felt unworthy to have Jesus in his home. Let Jesus simply give the command and the boy would be healed. The Centurion was a man under orders himself, and he in turn had many soldiers under him. If he gave a command, it would be obeyed. He did not have to go and carry it out in person. Could not Jesus do the same? 'But give the command and the boy will be healed'. His was faith indeed, and humility. When he heard the Centurion's message, Jesus turned to his followers and said, 'I tell you, nowhere, not even in Israel, have I found faith like this'.

Much doubt has been cast on the stories of Christ's miracles. Historians know that miracles have often been attributed to temporal leaders, such as rival Roman emperors, to indicate divine support, especially in the more 'superstitious' East of the Mediterranean world; but the fact that it was worth manufacturing miracles to lend support to an imperial propaganda campaign only shows that they were taken seriously, and why should that be so unless miracles had happened? They still do today. Doctors are often astonished by recoveries from diseases they had considered terminal. As for the story of the Centurion, it rings true to me for two reasons. First, the Centurion was a Roman, and when Luke adds the detail that he was friendly to the Jews and had built them a local synagogue, he is trying to minimise the foreignness of this man, a Roman of all people, who received such an accolade from Jesus. It would have been much easier just to have left this slightly embarrassing story out - especially for Matthew, the most 'Jewish' of the evangelists - if it had not been true and well remembered. Second, the Centurion's simple logic carries credibility. Here was a man used to giving and obeying orders. If he ordered something to be done, it would be done. It had better be. And it was.

I prayed then in an agony of grief for faith like the Centurion's. I pushed aside thoughts of the millions of starving and diseased children in distant lands and concentrated on my own loved one as I knelt by her unmade bed. Yet problems kept assailing me even as I prayed.

'Dear God, let her live. You surely cannot have given us such a lovely child only to let her die so soon or be horribly maimed'. But lots of lovely children do die or are maimed. Some indeed do not even have fourteen years of health to start with: they are born to a whole life of deformity and pain. Why? Can a God who is all-loving be all-mighty if he allows such suffering? But without suffering and pain, how would health and happiness be known, for without the contrast they could have no meaning? But why should God help Clare in particular and listen to the agonised prayer of this one set of parents in a world of billions? 'Without your Father's leave not a sparrow can fall to the ground', but that only means that God knows and does nothing. Or if there is life after death, is it wrong to pray for continuance of life on earth, especially if it could mean condemning a child to spend the rest of its days in pain or severely disabled in body or mind? No, it is not wrong. It cannot be. Clare must not die.

As I knelt by her bed I suddenly knew so clearly that I would find the strength to help Clare make the best of whatever abilities were left to her, and that I would love her as much as ever. Of course I had had my ambitions for her, as all parents do. She had been blessed with a good brain (if indeed intelligence is a blessing), and Mary and I had envisaged her perhaps following in our footsteps to Cambridge and a professional career. But none of this seemed important now. If Clare would only live, we would do our best to make her as happy and fulfilled as possible. For even Christ himself never said that it was better for any of the sick whom he healed to die, however wonderful the after-life might be. His compassion went out to them, and he was particularly sensitive to the loss of children. I was like Jairus, falling on my knees and begging Jesus to heal his only child, a twelve-year-old daughter, who was dying. 'Please, God', I prayed, 'let me have the faith of the Centurion, and do for my only child what you did for the daughter of Jairus'.

CHAPTER THREE

I had put the few things I had collected for Clare in a cheerful, brightly coloured duffel bag which she was fond of, and when Mary unpacked it at her bedside in the Trauma Unit we hardly dared look at each other for fear of breaking down. Clare liked to go to sleep listening to taped stories, her favourites being *Black Beauty, Kim,* the Mowgli stories from *The Jungle Book* and C.S. Lewis's tales of Narnia, but when we put one into the tape machine and laid it on the pillow by her ear, there was no flicker of recognition. It was just another mechanical noise like that of the ventilator's rhythmic inhalations and exhalations and the clicking of the banks of monitors above her head. The only sounds from Clare were the dreadful gurglings of the fluid collecting in her bruised chest. We then took her favourite sleeping companion, a once handsome but now rather mangy-looking and almost unrecognisable fluffy lion, and put him in the crook of her left arm, which was the only part of her that moved. But even dear old Leo could evoke no recognition or response and fell forlornly to the floor. It all seemed so very hopeless. From time to time the neurosurgeons came in, checked the charts and conferred with the nurses. They prised open Clare's black and swollen eyes and shone torches in them. Then they would pinch her very hard on her arms or legs and draw the sharp end of a key across the soles of her feet to check for reflexes, but only the left side responded. There was nothing at all from the right.

The head of the neurosurgical team that week-end was the Senior Registrar, Mr John Sutcliffe, a tall and intense-looking Yorkshireman who looked to be in his mid-thirties. At first he seemed rather austere, though obviously highly intelligent and experienced, but he was not a man to waste time with much small talk and he was evidently worried about Clare. He explained to me very clearly what the situation was. As young Dr Britto had said the previous night, although Clare's skull was fractured above the right eye, the force of the blow had flung the brain hard against the left front temple, and the swellings from both contusions were combining to create a dangerous level of pressure. But it was the damage to the left frontal lobe that was the greater danger. If it had been only the right side there would have been much less to worry about, as we apparently use relatively little of the right side of our brains. The left fronto-temporal area in a right-handed person is the one that does all the work, and the fact that Clare is very strongly right-handed and that side of her body was not responding at all was not good. 'We shall give her another CT scan in a little while,' said Mr Sutcliffe, 'and in the meantime we are administering a drug which has the effect of shrinking the brain and taking some of the pressure off the bruised areas. But we cannot do this for long, and if the pressure does not begin to come down soon I am afraid we shall have to operate and remove the damaged part of the left frontal lobe'.

We felt stunned when we heard this, and I felt my hand grasped tightly by Mary's. My friend Hughie Webb at St Thomas's had already warned me that they might need to operate to remove part of the skull to give the brain room to expand, but Mr Sutcliffe was talking about removing part of the brain itself. Would this really be necessary to reduce the pressure if it did not start coming down of its own accord? 'I am afraid so', he replied. 'Continued pressure would almost certainly mean that a piece of the brain has been damaged beyond recovery and it would have to be removed. But even if we have to do this, it needn't mean that Clare won't make a good recovery. The name of the operation, a lobotomy, sounds awful, I know, and it is not something we do except as a last resort to avoid the more serious and permanent damage that would occur if we did nothing. But I have done over twenty-five of them myself, and some patients have recovered so well that after a few months it would have taken detailed psychometric tests to detect any impairment at all. To all intents and purposes they have been 100% normal again and no-one who did not know what had happened would ever guess. It all depends on the amount and location of the damage. But an operation may not be necessary at all. Only time will tell. We shall see what happens during the course of the day'.

Mary and I discussed whether or not to tell any of our relations or friends about Clare's accident but decided against it. There seemed no point in upsetting them at this stage when we had no idea of the likely outcome. Our closest relatives were our two elderly mothers - mine with severe Alzheimer's disease in a nursing home in the North of England, Mary's recently widowed and living in Cambridge - and Mary's brother, himself a doctor at the Addenbrooke's hospital in Cambridge but spending a few months at a hospital in New Zealand at that time. Besides, we felt we wanted to be alone with Clare without distractions. Nothing else mattered. We did, however, have two visitors early in the afternoon, and though they were both unknown to us, they were very welcome.

One was Vicky, the fourteen-year-old whom the nurses and the helicopter doctor had told us about. She had been in a similar state to Clare only a few weeks ago, indeed considerably worse. She had had to undergo two of the operations which Clare could now be facing, and she had had pneumonia too. Now she appeared in a wheel-chair with the happiest parents imaginable, and she needed the chair only because she had smashed a leg very badly and it was still in metal clamps sticking out at crazy angles. Mentally she was fine, and though shy she gave us a lovely smile before chatting away to the nurses, who were thrilled to see her. Her father told me they had heard about Clare and wondered whether or not to come in. We were so glad they did. It gave us great hope. I have to confess, though, that I felt a momentary pang of envy, which I suppressed with disgust. God grant that we should be as fortunate with Clare as they had been with their lovely daughter, but if that could not be, only let her live.

Our other visitor was a police Inspector from Bow Street Police Station. It was a detachment of officers from Bow Street who had been in the van behind the bus when Clare jumped off and fell. They had seen the whole thing, given first aid, then commandeered the passing St John ambulance which had rushed her into the Westminster Hospital. Inspector Allison could not have been kinder. He was coming off duty and 'the lads' had asked him to call in and see how Clare was. I suppose many of them were fathers themselves and their hearts had clearly gone out to Clare because both the hospitals, first the Westminster, then the London, had had regular calls from Bow Street to see how she was. And now Inspector Chris Allison had come himself to ask if he could do anything to help and to tell us exactly what had happened. He had the full story from P.C. Paul Anstey, who had tended Clare at the scene of the accident, and P.C. Peter Scopes who had managed to identify her and trace us.

Mary and I were very touched by his kindness, and as I was sitting by Clare's bedside three days later I wrote a letter to the London *Evening Standard,* which was published under the headline 'Give the police a break'. There is always so much adverse publicity about the police, and it was particularly bad at that time because of a shocking incident where an innocent man had been arrested and beaten up. But while it is of course right that bad things should be exposed, the condemnation is disproportionate to the praise that is given for the infinitely greater number of good things, and I wanted to redress the balance a bit in the light of my own experience. The letter read as follows:

'With the police receiving so much bad publicity - in general and, more recently, in particular over the mistreatment of an innocent suspect - I must say I wish that more publicity could be given to the good things they do, which is the rule rather than the exception.

Last Saturday my 14-year-old daughter was severely injured in an accident and suffered considerable brain damage. The police were superb. It was not only that they helped get her into hospital very quickly, traced us and rushed us there, but they then rang the hospital every hour throughout the night to see how she was and every four hours for the next two critical days until her life was out of danger. An Inspector from Bow Street also visited us in the hospital - not because there was any criminal aspect to the case (it had been a pure accident; my daughter had slipped off the platform of a moving bus) but purely out of kindness.

In any large organisation there will be failures and especially in a police force which every day sees the worst of human nature. But when it comes to what is typical, my experience of the last few days is what counts - an experience which must be multiplied a thousand times every day but is rarely publicised. I feel very proud and grateful to live in a city and country that has a police force with the combination of professionalism and humanity that I have witnessed in the last few days'.

We had seen the Inspector in a private room and when we returned to the Trauma Unit we found Clare being attended to by Linda, the thoracic physiotherapist. Linda was pleased with the way the fluid was coming up, but despite the convulsions in the chest there was still little reaction from Clare's limbs, particularly on the right side, and the brain pressure monitor kept going sky-high. What on earth was going on behind those bruised and battered eyes? It was certainly good news that Linda was now much less worried about Clare's chest, but what about the brain, the intelligence, the personality? What about the real 'Clare'?

'I'm sending you two off to bed' came a voice from behind us. It was Sandra, the Sister, as she marked Clare's chart. 'You can't do much for Clare at present, but you will be able to do a lot later on. You mustn't exhaust yourselves so that you are useless when you are really needed.'

'Perhaps one of us could stay and the other go and rest for a bit, so Clare always has one of us with her', ventured Mary.

'That's a good idea for later, when she is conscious of your presence', said Sandra, 'but for now I'm packing you both off to have something to eat and a little rest.'

'You'll phone us at once if there is any change.'

'Of course I will. I know where you are. Don't worry, she's in good hands.' She certainly was.

We had a bite to eat in the canteen, then went to rest on the bed for a couple of hours. I set an alarm clock, but it was unnecessary. Though we were both so tired that we fell into a sleep that seemed miles deep, I woke up of my own accord just before the clock was due to go off. For a moment I wondered where I was, then suddenly I realised that I was waking to a nightmare, not escaping one. Mary was still asleep. I went out quietly to the kitchen and made us both a pot of tea before wakening her. Then we showered, changed into fresh clothes and went back to the Trauma Unit.

It was about 7.30 in the evening and the day shift was preparing to hand over to the night staff. Sandra greeted us and introduced us to her colleagues coming on duty, Jan and Lynn.

'Clare is just the same', Sandra replied to our unspoken question. 'Mr Sutcliffe came in at one stage and asked me to prepare her for theatre but then changed his mind. He is still hoping that the brain pressure will drop sufficiently to avoid an operation. We are still giving her the brain-reducing drug and she will have another CT scan a bit later.'

It seemed to me that Sandra had thought an operation would be needed and had been surprised by the surgeon's decision to leave it a bit longer. Mary and I looked at each other and her hand reached out for mine. We had clung to the hope that there would be no need to operate. We had told the police Inspector that, and had come to believe it. The thought of removing a piece of the brain was too horrific.

'But do *you* think an operation will be necessary after all?' I challenged Sandra. 'Mr Sutcliffe seemed so confident that it wouldn't.'

I should not have asked this question of Sandra, I knew, but she did not try to evade it. 'I must say I did think it would be necessary, but try not to worry. They will decide later, and there is no immediate danger. They won't do anything they don't have to. But the pressure has got to come down.'

We sat down by Clare's bed, kissed her and stroked her arms and legs. There was no response, but she was certainly a better colour than she had been in the Westminster when her body-temperature had been so low. The nurses had also cleaned her up as well as they could without disturbing all the equipment, and she looked very peaceful. But her poor face was pear-shaped, her jaw and neck hugely swollen as though her whole face had sagged, her eyes bruised, swollen and tightly shut. Tubes and wires seemed to come out of everywhere, ventilating her, feeding her, emptying her bladder, infusing antibiotics and the drug to try to reduce the brain pressure which was being monitored through the dreadful metal aerial protruding through her skull. We could not take our eyes off that monitor, willing it to come down when it ran up into the thirties and forties, willing it to stay down when it fell below twenty; but that was less and less often and we began to fear the worst.

The meticulous change-over from day to night staff took about half an hour. The charts of the Unit's three patients were studied while still being up-dated every five or ten minutes, details of the treatments discussed in low voices and questions asked and answered. It was all superbly professional. But it made us feel even more helpless. We tried to keep talking to Clare and stroking her arms and legs, to try and let her know that we were with her, but still we watched in vain for even a flicker of consciousness of our presence.

The evening dragged on until about 9 o'clock, when Mr Sutcliffe and two of his colleagues came in again, examined the charts and checked on the arrangements for the brain scan.

He examined Clare and produced an encouraging jerk in her limbs by nipping her hard or scratching the soles of her feet with a key, but the response was still minimal on the right side.

'How is she doing?' I asked, really meaning 'Will she need an operation?'

'We are going to have her scanned again, then we'll know more,' he replied, adding 'Now there's just time for you two to get a bite to eat before the canteen closes, so why not take a little break while the scan is being done. It will be an hour at least before she's finished, and there's no danger: it's just an X-ray of the brain.'

In the canteen we saw the wife of the very sick man in the far bed in the Trauma Unit. He was a big, fine-looking man in his fifties. Like Clare, he was wired up to the full resuscitation machinery and totally unconscious. He had been there when Clare arrived, but so far we had not done more than exchange greetings with his wife. Now her family had gone and we found her on her own having a coffee and a sandwich. For a moment we hesitated. We really wanted to be alone with our thoughts and perhaps she did too, but when she noticed us it was clear that she would like some company so we joined her and exchanged stories.

Hers was appalling. Her husband, Len, was a crane-driver on the Canary Wharf building site in London's docklands, which were only a few minutes drive from the Hospital. He had been crossing a road on the site at some traffic lights which were not working. Someone had put up a sign of some sort sticking out into the road, and as Len edged out to see if it was clear to cross, a site bus sped past and knocked him flying, causing terrible internal damage. The private ambulance used on the site had been called, and as he was being put into it writhing in pain, the London Hospital's helicopter happened to be passing overhead and descended to see if they could help. It had the doctor on board, could have had Len on resuscitation immediately and in the hospital ten minutes later, but incredibly - and worryingly - the helicopter was waved away. Two hours later the ambulance dumped Mr Davies in Casualty reception at the London without any notes, and it was only when he regained consciousness and began screaming with pain that they realised how urgent his case was. Something like three hours had been lost, and Len was very ill indeed. Yet when Mrs Davies rang the contractor on the site to say what had happened, his sole reaction had been a blasphemous complaint that his other skilled crane-driver had cut his hand and they hadn't got a spare. We were to hear more of the goings-on at Canary Wharf later from one of the Trauma Unit nurses who had been seconded there for six months, and it left a lot to be desired - and investigated.

On our way back to the Unit we stopped at the hospital's W.H.

Smith shop, which is open from about 8 a.m. to 10 p.m. and has everything from stationery, newspapers, magazines and cards to a whole range of things to eat and drink, toiletries and so on. We had noticed that the nurses and visiting doctors loved biscuits and chocolates and would often send out for some with much counting of coins. So we bought a big box of Quality Street chocolates and some Penguin chocolate biscuits, and continued to buy something of the sort for the staff every day, much to their amusement and enjoyment. Relatives of patients should always remember: nurses and doctors love chocolates and cakes and biscuits, and because they are on their feet burning up energy most of the day they can eat them without the problems of physical inflation that beset more sedentary occupations.

As Clare was not yet back from being scanned we left the comestibles in the Unit and went down to the hospital's little chapel on the ground floor, which was open all the time. There was no one there, but a lamp was burning over the plain, wooden altar. A crucifix hung on the opposite wall next to a stained glass window, which we later discovered had been made by a nun who was part of the hospital's Chaplaincy. The only other ornament was an impressionist tapestry of a sunrise on the other wall, yet this sparsely furnished Chapel was strangely welcoming as we knelt and prayed. Then as we sat for a while without talking, the whirling kaleidoscope of my thoughts suddenly resolved itself into a picture of a little old lady, long dead, who had lived next door to us nearly twenty years ago, long before Clare was born.

We had been married only a couple of years then and lived in what estate agents would call a 'bijou Victorian cottage' at the village of Thames Ditton, opposite Hampton Court Palace. We had stretched our borrowing powers to the limit in buying it for £14,000, but it was modernised to the extent of central heating, an internal bathroom and a garage. Our neighbour, Mrs Eley, well on in her seventies then, was not modernised at all. Her house still had an outside lavatory, though a door had been knocked through to it from the kitchen so that she did not have to go out in the rain and cold to attend to nature. But why did I think of her now?

We had not long moved into our house there when I had to face a series of fairly serious spinal operations, and for several months between and after them I was able to convalesce at home, though needing to spend quite a lot of time horizontal and wearing a great plastic breastplate when I was vertical. Mrs Eley used to make my lunch and generally 'mother' me while Mary was at work. She was an angel. Thanks to her marvellous pies and roasts and apple dumplings I soon began to use less tight holes on the straps of my corset, which was just as well as I had looked like a survivor of Belsen when I first came out of hospital. But just as welcome as the marvellous lunches was the spiritual food that Mrs Eley supplied, usually quite unconsciously.

When the old lady, as the Salvationists say, was 'promoted to glory' a few years ago, I have no doubt that the pearly gates were wide open to receive her. From a virtually nineteenth-century country upbringing in Norfolk where her father had been head gardener at a stately home she had joined the Salvation Army and exchanged the pure Norfolk air for the foetid slums of the East End, exactly the area that the London Hospital served. Of course she caught every illness going, but she survived and stuck to her vocation. She used to describe how she and the other girls in training would return to their barracks exhausted both physically and mentally after a day's work in the most appalling conditions. Once, she said, she was so hungry and cold, but there was a cockroach in the soup and she was sick, and that night she felt that she could stand no more and would have to give up. But as she lay on her bunk wondering how on earth she could face another day, the girl in the bunk above happened to drop a box of biblical 'promises', which fluttered down all over her like blossom from a cherry tree. This, plus the Captain's idiosyncratic method of saying 'goodnight' as she went round and turned the lights out, gave her fresh hope, for instead of 'goodnight' the indomitable Captain used to cry cheerfully, 'Keep believing, keep believing!' And she did.

Mrs Eley was a marvellous person. The little houses where we lived then were in semi-detached pairs. Mrs Eley's house was separated from ours by our two gardens (which were at the sides of each pair of houses), and in the house which adjoined hers on the other side lived a rather rough family whose rows were famous in the neighbourhood for both the volume of sound and the ripeness of the vocabulary. They had a teenage son who was always getting into trouble. He used to go out collecting with a charity box devoted to the principle that charity begins at home, and he was forever joy-riding in cars or, on the river, speed-boats. Instead of putting him in the army, teaching him a trade and letting him drive tanks at full speed over

Salisbury Plain, he was put into a remand home to learn even more wickedness from the far tougher cases who were there. But Mrs Eley never lost faith in him. She wrote to him every day while he was in prison, and when he came out she was the first person he went to see. Mary, going over to Mrs Eley's one day, came back without knocking: through the window she had seen her and this young man kneeling together in prayer by the hearth. 'Keep believing!' That is why I thought of dear Mrs Eley now.

When we went upstairs again Clare was just back from radiography and the tension in the room was tangible as we went in. No-one was bothering about the monitor figures any longer. The scans were up against the illuminated screen by the door, and Mr Sutcliffe and Dr Britto were examining them closely.

'I'm afraid we shall have to operate', Mr Sutcliffe told us without preamble. 'The pressure is not coming down, and if we do not intervene surgically soon your daughter could suffer irreparable damage. I'm very sorry, but I promise you it is absolutely essential.' He then showed me the scans. 'That', he said, pointing to a vaguely darker patch on the temple, is the area of damaged cells that has to be removed. It is unfortunate, as I said before, that the damage is on the left side, but with luck - and I must stress that the scans are not so accurate that I can be sure - it looks as though the damage may have missed the speech area'.

'And is that the only damaged area?' I asked.

'I don't know', he replied. 'The bump on the right temple where the skull is fractured may not be very dangerous but what we cannot tell is how much contusion and bleeding there might be deeper in the brain. It would not show up on the scan. But children are better off than adults in this respect, because there are fissures in the brain which have not yet closed up at Clare's age, and these allow the blood from internal bleeding to escape to the surface without building up more pressure deep inside. All I know for sure at this stage is that we have to do something urgently about the contusion on the frontal lobe, and I must ask you to give me permission to operate at once. I have postponed it as long as I dare. To postpone it any longer would carry far greater risks than to operate. I promise you it is for the best.'

Mary and I looked at each other, then at Mr Sutcliffe, and I nodded. We trusted him, and he knew it.

'I shall do my best,' he said. 'I won't say "Try not to worry", but

I will say "Remember the young lady I hear you saw today, Vicky". She was even more seriously damaged than Clare. She needed two operations, not one, and look at her now. Admittedly she has done exceptionally well, but while I can't promise anything for Clare, there is a reasonable chance that any permanent damage will be small.' Then turning to the staff he said, 'Prepare Clare for theatre at once, please', and we were ushered out to the ITU waiting room, where a nurse soon arrived with a cup of tea. Mercifully the waiting room was otherwise empty. We did not feel we could face anyone else.

By now it was after midnight, but my friend Hughie Webb from St Thomas's had told me to ring at any time of the day or night, particularly if they decided to operate. I now did so, and he confirmed that they were doing the right thing.

'You must sign the consent form, Peter', he said, 'and let them go ahead. If the pressure is not going down after a whole day, they must operate otherwise there will be permanent disability for certain. If the pressure is allowed to go on too long, the cerebral cortex becomes affected, which means that all Clare's motor functions could be permanently impaired. In fact, it is a matter of life and death. They are operating to save her life. You must not hesitate to sign the form.'

I assured Hughie at once that I trusted the surgeons here and would certainly sign the form, but I still did not fully understand why they could not just remove a piece of the skull to relieve the pressure rather than removing a piece of the brain itself.

'The answer, Peter, is that that piece of brain is evidently so badly damaged that it is useless. If it is just mush, it has to be cleared away. But from all you say your surgeon sounds reasonably confident that the damage has missed the main speech areas. It is terrible, I know, but you must trust them and let them go ahead. Clare could not be in better hands. The London is superb for this kind of thing.'

I felt reassured by talking to Hughie, not because we had really doubted that the operation was necessary but because it was good to tell someone who is not only a very dear friend but also an expert neurologist himself. As before, he made me promise to ring him at any time if I needed him, and he would himself check with the hospital in the morning if he had not heard anything. I then went back to the waiting room, and I had scarcely finished telling Mary what Hughie had said than we were asked to come across to the Unit. As we crossed the landing, we saw Clare, her bed festooned with all her equipment and monitors, being wheeled once again through the double doors into the operating corridor. Dr Britto was waiting for us in the Unit and had the consent form ready for me to sign. I signed it at once, but then asked him to explain briefly once more what they were going to do. Though clearly in a hurry to go and scrub up to assist in theatre, he nevertheless answered our questions kindly and clearly, then he had no sooner left the room than he popped his head in again and told us to go and lie down for a bit. It was half past one in the morning, and the operation would be at least two hours.

We took his advice and went back to James Hora House. The sharp early morning air felt nice as we walked across the courtyard but made us conscious of our weariness, so having set the alarm clock once more we collapsed on our beds and were soon in a deep sleep of mental and physical exhaustion. As before I woke up just before the alarm clock went off, and by 3.30 we were back at the Unit to see what was happening. But Clare was still in theatre, so we took up our stations on the two stacking chairs, the red and the blue, where we had sat while Clare was having the head-bolt inserted the previous night. They were just outside the double doors leading to the operating theatres, so we were as near as possible to her. We talked little. What was there to say? Mary made us a cup of tea at one stage, but more for something to do than because we were thirsty. Each time the doors opened we looked anxiously to see if Clare or her surgeon were coming, and at last, about half past four, Mr Sutcliffe appeared. As I rose to greet him and looked at his face, I knew before he spoke that it had gone as well as it could. He was obviously terribly tired, but the look of relief on his face was unmistakable.

'Clare will be out in a few minutes', he said, 'and when they have sorted her out you will be able to see her. It went as well as I could have hoped. We have removed the damaged area, and providing there is nothing more sinister which we cannot see deep inside, she has a good chance of recovery.'

Mary and I clutched each other's hand and felt a great wave of relief sweeping over us. When I told Mr Sutcliffe that I had read the relief in his face even before he had spoken, he smiled, but warned us that although he was pleased with what he had seen so far, the next twenty-four hours would be critical, for only then would they be able to tell if the damage had been confined to the area he had dealt with.

Clare was still very seriously ill, and there was no knowing to what extent she would recover her faculties or even any certainty that she would survive. But so far, so good. The operation had gone as well as could have been hoped, and we should be able to see her shortly.

Clare herself emerged through the double doors a few minutes later and was wheeled rapidly into the Trauma Unit. There were so many people round her that we could hardly see her, but Lynn, the Trauma nurse who was looking after her that night, told us that she would call us as soon as they had settled Clare back. Then the anaesthetist, Dr Jo Challons, had a reassuring word with us, and young Dr Britto gave us a cheerful smile as he passed on his way to some other emergency in another ward. It is hard to praise them adequately without sounding either extravagant or sentimental, but the fact is that we felt we were among people of the very highest quality, combining the utmost professionalism with humanity and dedication. You could feel the pride and *esprit de corps* everywhere. It was very impressive, very reassuring, and really rather humbling.

Mr Sutcliffe's 'shortly' turned out to be a seemingly endless hour and a half, for it was about 6 o'clock in the morning when we were finally allowed in to see Clare. There were even more things sticking out of her now. Her forehead and the top of her head were completely swathed in bandages, which were fairly bloody in parts, and she now had a drainage tube leading from the back of her head in addition to the pressure-monitoring bolt protruding from the centre. Lynn explained that the drain was to get rid of blood from the surface of the brain only, and was standard procedure. Then there were all the other tubes and wires, the drips into neck and arm, a blood-oxygen monitor on her finger, taps for injections on her leg, the catheter and tube for urine, the electrocardiogram terminals on her chest, the ventilator over her mouth and various other tubes down her nose. She seemed very peaceful and somehow a long way away. We sat beside her and stroked her limbs as before, but this time without having to watch the pressure monitor so desperately as it was now recording nil. Lynn, who was 'specialing' Clare, and Jan, who was looking after Len Davies, were constantly busy, giving injections, checking monitors, marking up charts, sometimes helping each other when it needed two people to perform some task and taking turns to tend the third patient, the elderly lady in the far corner who was not on ventilation and not as critical as the other two. In the following days and nights we would get to know these and the other nurses well, and they were without exception lovely people. I kept on thinking how proud I should be if Clare were to recover completely and become a nurse in a Unit like this.

CHAPTER FOUR

About 7.30 the day staff came in, Sandra and Nick, and began their careful take-over routine with Jan and Lynn, though not without enjoying a chocolate biscuit first and complimenting their provider on his choice. I felt ridiculously pleased to have done something, however trivial, to show some appreciation to the staff and resolved that they would not lack for further supplies as long as Clare was there.

It was Sandra who was looking after Clare again as she had done the previous day, and when I mentioned that she had been right that Clare would need the operation she smiled and said 'I've been doing this job quite a long time. But don't you worry. Remember Vicky was worse than Clare.' Then she ordered us to go and have some breakfast. 'You'll need all your strength as the days go by', she added cheerfully.

Having not eaten much for forty-eight hours Mary and I found we were suddenly very hungry, and when we went over to the canteen and saw huge trays of hot bacon, eggs and sausages - and young doctors and nurses cheerfully mopping up the delicious cholesterol - we did ourselves proud, and felt much better for it. The only problem was the amazing complexity of the tea and coffee machine. In my unintelligent state I remember staring stupidly at the Filtrona with my sachet of tea in my hand and not the least idea what to do with it. The trick was to insert the sachet into a vertical drawer at the right of the machine after putting a cup on the stand underneath, but being notoriously useless with gadgetry I had to watch a young nurse operating the next one before I discovered this. I felt an absurd sense of triumph when eventually I had managed to get a couple of cups of tea, and at least I had made Mary smile for the first time since Clare's accident.

I then remembered that I must move the car, which I had been able to leave over the week-end right outside the front entrance of the hospital on Whitechapel Road, but during week-days this was a bus-lane so I had to move it before 8.30. As the immediate vicinity of the hospital is all a controlled zone with parking limited to a few meter-spaces, I had to go about half a mile before I found a side-street where I could leave the car all day, and I did so with some trepidation as I had heard terrible stories of cars, or at least their wheels, disappearing without trace in that 'rough' area. But as usual these stories were exaggerated. I certainly had no trouble at all in the next three weeks while the car was left in neighbouring streets day and night, nor did I see any 'suspicious characters' when I was walking back to the hospital. I just felt refreshed by the morning air and the exercise.

When I got back to the Trauma Unit I found Mary fixing a tape into Clare's small recorder and putting it on the pillow beside her. It was David Davies reading *Black Beauty,* one of Clare's (and our) favourites. The poignancy of the story and the elegant simplicity of the style put it, for me at least, in the very front rank of animal books. Its Victorian author, herself crippled in her youth and in pain for much of her life, knew only too well what suffering was, and her compassion for the often harsh lives of working horses is not sentimental but real. I thought she would have been pleased to think of it being read so beautifully on the pillow of another injured child, and though Clare seemed to me still too deeply unconscious to be able to receive anything even subconsciously, Sandra felt that it could help to stimulate her mind as it was slowly reawakening.

A few minutes later the telephone rang on the desk and I heard Sandra telling someone that Clare was satisfactory after the operation and there was no cause for concern. I wondered who it could be, then Sandra told us it was Bow Street police. Inspector Allison's men were all loyally rooting for Clare and had apparently rung twice during the night. We were very touched by their continuing kindness and concern, and it was now that I began to think that I should write to the papers about it.

We decided that we must make some telephone calls of our own. Mary went first and rang her office. She is a partner of a small firm of solicitors in Greenwich, and the colleague to whom she spoke, the other lady partner, offered at once to take over Mary's work. She knew only too well what Mary was going through. She had nearly lost her husband not long before from a rare type of blood cancer, which had needed some very unpleasant treatment before it was brought under control. Then Mary rang our 'daily', Mrs Dolding, who would be alarmed to find no-one at home and see the message that Mary had left for me when the police had called, as I had forgotten to take it away when I went home to collect our clean clothes. We also asked Mrs Dolding not to answer the phone, so she would not have to make excuses if asked where we were. I had left an answering machine on, and we could pick up messages later from that. For the time being we wanted neither to worry friends and relations nor be bothered with them ourselves, at least not until these critical twenty-four hours were over.

When Mary returned I went to make my own calls, first of course to Hughie Webb to let him know what had happened, but I could not get him. I then rang one of my business colleagues, also a very dear friend, and he, like Mary's partner, immediately offered to look after everything for as long as was necessary. He himself had been through a worrying time with his own daughter, who had gone through a terrible period of depression for no apparent reason, for she is a lovely girl, attractive, kind and with everything to live for. Happily she is now over it, thanks to a course of drugs which corrected what was evidently a chemical imbalance of some sort in the brain. But it is somehow harder to come to terms with mental than physical illness, despite the fact that no force of will can create missing enzymes in the brain any more than it can create insulin for a diabetic.

Finally I rang our Vicar, Clifford Knowles, another dear friend. His parish is in the decayed cotton-town of Heywood in Lancashire, a long way from London, but I was born there and we visit it about every month or six weeks to see my mother, who is in a nursing home in nearby Rochdale, famous as the home of Gracie Fields and the Co-operative Movement. When I was left a little terraced house by my mother's brother a few years ago I kept it on as somewhere to stay and take my mother out to when we came to visit her. She has been suffering from senile dementia for ten years, but happily she still just about recognises us and is not unhappy or violent as so many victims of Alzheimer's disease are. She used to love to go to church with us on our week-end visits and see my father's cousin Billy, who has sung in the choir for seventy years. Sadly she is not well enough to be able to sit through a service now, but the Vicar visits her at Leighton House, where she is beautifully cared for, and we go to Holy Communion on the Sunday mornings before driving back to London after spending the Saturdays with her.

St Luke's is a tall and very handsome example of Victorian Gothic at its most elegant. The old Bishop of Manchester used to call it 'Heywood Cathedral', but these days it is as hard to fill as to heat, even for an incumbent of Clifford's calibre. There is nevertheless a solid corps of regulars, and it was a great joy to us when Clare and our nineteen-year-old goddaughter, Frances, were confirmed there the previous year. I wanted my friend's prayers for Clare now more than ever. He spoke so kindly and encouragingly that I found myself choking to keep the emotion of the last forty-eight hours under control, and as soon as I had put the receiver down I hurried to the hospital chapel, which was empty, wept like a child and begged God to help Clare. Somehow I felt sure she would live and I dedicated myself to making the best possible life for her, whatever disabilities she might have.

Though I washed my face in cold water before returning to the Trauma Unit, Mary could see that I had been upset and put her hand into mine without a word. Men are supposed to be the stronger sex, but they are not. It is women who bear the pain of childbirth and have the emotional strength and self-control at times like this when nothing active can be done to ease a pain. I would cheerfully have gone over the top of a trench or given my own life to save Clare, but when the need is for passive patience women are generally much better at coping with it.

About 10 o'clock Hughie Webb phoned through to the Trauma Unit. He had already spoken to Clare's surgeon, and I could tell by his voice that he was relieved by what he had heard, though he reiterated that today would be critical. He also told me to be sure that Mary and I got some rest, as we should be no help to Clare if we cracked up ourselves. It was not the first time we had been told this in the last forty-eight hours, and while there was no way that we were going to leave Clare alone today, we decided to take it in turns to have a rest so that one of us would always be with her.

It was a long day, but one of constant activity around Clare. The neurosurgical team came in several times to examine the charts, confer with the nurses and examine Clare's reflexes, but for a long time there was evidently little response in her eyes when they managed to raise the swollen lids and shine a torch on them, and there was still little or nothing from her limbs, particularly on the right. Even when Linda came in and Clare went into paroxysms of coughing as she struck her back to loosen the phlegm and Sandra inserted the suction tubes that made her retch, no hand shot up to push her away and only the left leg bent and flexed itself. But we were worried unnecessarily by the astonishing amount of fluid that was coming up.

Linda quickly reassured us that it was excellent to see the lungs clearing so well now, and she felt that it would not be too long before Clare started to regain consciousness.

By midday even the stoical Mary was looking exhausted, and I sent her off to have a bite to eat and a rest, promising to wake her instantly if there was any change. She came back about 3 o'clock, then I went over to the hostel. I bought myself a sandwich on the way, made a cup of tea in the kitchen, then went out like a light until the alarm clock woke me at 5.30, for this time, unusually, my internal clock had not woken me as it generally did just before the electric one.

I arrived back at the Unit to find Mr Sutcliffe and Dr Britto with Clare. They were pleased that the brain pressure was staying well below danger levels and were now cautiously hopeful that there was no more sinister bruising deeper inside. They seemed a bit disappointed that Clare's right side was still not responding much yet, but it was early days. It was reassuring to be taken so fully into their confidence instead of being shooed out of the room whenever doctors came in and kept in the dark, as used to be the practice when I was a boy: indeed the whole system of visiting then seemed to be designed to ensure that doctors were never troubled by relatives, and relatives had to suffer in ignorance as the nurses were forbidden to say anything themselves.

When Sandra went over to assist Nick with Len, who was beginning to regain consciousness, I quietly emptied a plastic bag full of chocolate bars and biscuits onto her desk and pretended innocence when she noticed them. The surgeons, physios and nurses had all been dipping so eagerly into the Quality Street that the commissariat needed replenishing, and there was much appreciative absorption of calories when the night staff came on for the changeover.

Mary and I took it in turns to go for supper in the canteen, where I could not help smiling at the heaps of chips that the doctors, nurses and other staff were tucking away. It was not that there were no so-called 'health foods': there was a vast and rather dusty heap of muesli bars, and a hot vegetarian meal with lots of pulse and soya-beans. But the most popular offering with the longest queue was steak and kidney pie served with a suggestion of cabbage and a veritable mountain of French fries. I had it myself and it was delicious.

As usual when I returned to Clare I glanced anxiously at the brain-pressure monitor before anything else, but happily it was still moving in a fairly stable band comfortably below the danger level. Poor Mary looked so tired and said she did not feel like eating, but I made her promise to have something in the canteen, and when she returned, having also succumbed to the steak and kidney pie, she was much better. In the meantime I had had a visitor, the hospital Chaplain. It turned out that he had been in the Chaplaincy at St Thomas's before coming to the London, and had been great friends there with my friend Hughie Webb. Hughie had now rung him and asked him to visit us. I was so sorry that Mary had missed him, but he promised to come again.

It must be a very difficult job being a Chaplain, seeing so much sadness, trying to comfort the dying and the bereaved when their world seems to be disintegrating, sometimes finding faith but sometimes anger and even insult. In the days that followed I got to know Peter Cowell quite well, and I soon understood why Hughie had been so sorry when he left St Thomas's. He had a firm but unobtrusive sincerity and faith that were almost tangible, yet far from radiating an air of embarrassment as so many clerics unfortunately do, he had the unaffected and natural approachability that I imagine the first disciples must have had, down-to-earth types who did not pretend to understand the incomprehensible but knew that they followed One who did and to whose example they could strive but not attain. He was such another man as our Vicar in Lancashire, and if only some of the higher echelons of the Church hierarchy could emulate some of these humbler priests working in the field, the Church of England would be a healthier and less inadequate force for good in an age and society that desperately need some moral leadership.

I remember telling the Chaplain how wonderfully Clare was being cared for, and how impressed I was by the quality and dedication of the young nurses who were attending her. I also told him what I had thought earlier, that if Clare were to recover fully and were to chose to go in for nursing with a group of young people of this calibre, I should be the proudest father in the world. 'You must be the proudest father in the world whatever happens', he replied. 'You must be the proudest father right now.' It was a wonderful thing to say. I looked at my poor Clare, so battered and bruised, and I loved her even more than I had ever done before.

When the Chaplain had gone I again thought of all my dreams for Clare, just as I had done when I knelt by her bed at home the previous day, which seemed more like a year ago. She was a bright child, particularly keen on the sciences rather than the arts at school but forever with her nose in a book or reading a play at home. I had been able to give her a good start in life, and by the time she was ten she had travelled to more countries than I had when I was thirty. I had been the classical working-class lad who had won a free place to the local Grammar School, one of those great social levellers that I can never forgive a Labour government's hypocrisy for destroying while leaving the public schools alone (with quite a few of the Labour ministers' children in them). I had won a scholarship from there to Cambridge, where I met Mary, and we cherished a dream that Claire might perhaps follow us there. But what was really important in life? To be happy and fulfilled, and that means giving rather than receiving and doing your best with the abilities you have. Yes, I was proud of the Clare that had been and I should be just as proud of the Clare that was to be, whether the future restored her to her full powers or confined her to a wheel-chair or left her somewhere in between. If only she could regain the use of her limbs and work in a stable among her beloved horses, she could be happy and fulfilled doing it to the best of her abilities. I thought of the lovely old hymn we used to sing at school: 'Who sweeps a room as for Thy laws, Makes that and the action fine'. And Christ himself was born in a stable.

These are the trains of thought that occupied my mind as Mary and I sat with Clare that Monday evening until they were interrupted by the arrival of Linda for another session of lung-clearing. Clare's eyes were still tightly shut - indeed one was so bruised that it could not have opened if Clare had been awake - but there was definitely more response now from her limbs. As the violent expectorations convulsed her once more, her left arm as well as her left leg began to move, and its movements were not just automatic reflexes.

This time her left hand did wave about as though deliberately, albeit drunkenly, trying to push the tubes away.

'That's a good sign', said Linda, exchanging a nod of approval with Angela and Pat, the night staff, and when I took hold of Clare's hand I distinctly felt it pushing against me. There was even a bit of movement on the right side now, and when Linda scratched the bare sole of Clare's right foot, we rejoiced to see her right knee bend - not much, but the reflex was clearly there. Angela then prised Clare's less swollen eye open and shone her torch on the pupil. 'That's better too', she said, and when Mr Sutcliffe and his team came in about 10 o'clock to see how Clare was doing, he was clearly encouraged too. He confirmed that the reflexes were discernible now on both sides, though very feeble so far on the right, but most of all he was relieved to see that the brain pressure graph had continued to remain below the danger line. It had now been sufficiently stable for long enough for him to be reasonably confident that there was no serious bruising deeper in the brain that had not showed up on the scan. We were coming towards the end of the critical twenty-four-hour post-operative period, and provided nothing abnormal occurred in the night Clare's life was out of immediate danger.

Mary and I felt a wave of relief pouring over us, and when Mr Sutcliffe had finished his discussions with the nursing staff, I followed him out into the corridor on impulse and asked him if I could shake his hand. He looked taken aback for a moment and hesitated before doing so. 'There are many things that could go wrong yet', he said, 'so don't get too excited. We seem to have done enough to sort out the brain pressure problem, but there is always the danger of an infection. And we have no way of telling yet to what extent she may be impaired. You could have to face a very different life for her in the future than she has had in the past.'

'Don't worry', I replied. 'Mary and I understand that, and we are prepared for whatever we may have to face. But your courage and skill have saved her life from the immediate threat and given her the best possible chance of a good recovery. That is why I wanted to shake your hand, not because I think it will be plain sailing from now on to a full recovery.'

Mr Sutcliffe relaxed when I said this and became less austere. 'Be prepared for the worst', he said, 'but hope for the best. You saw Vicky and how well she recovered. But Vicky is a real star. It's not always like that, and we simply don't know yet with Clare. All I can say, as before, is "so far, so good". Anyway she is beginning to regain consciousness now and we may even be able to get her off the ventilator tomorrow.' Then he added the instruction we had heard so often already. 'Now make sure you and your wife get some sleep tonight. You will need all your strength as Clare begins to come round and we can start the rehabilitation programme.'

Mary and I then took it in turns to make some telephone calls, mine to Hughie Webb and our Vicar, Mary's to her colleague at the office, then we sat with Clare till about 1.30 in the morning. By now Clare's left hand was constantly moving towards the ventilator or trying to pull at her catheter tube, feebly still but with semi-conscious purpose. We kept holding the hand down and thrilled to feel it pushing against us so deliberately. Then the staff shared a pot of tea with us, and though we were unwilling to tear ourselves away they urged us kindly but firmly to get some rest, promising as always to let us know at once if there was anything wrong. We obeyed, and when I bent to kiss Clare good night and felt the pressure of her feebly waving hand I whispered in her ear, 'Keep it up, Clare love. Come back to us soon.'

CHAPTER FIVE

I resumed my usual habit of waking myself up just before the alarm clock went off at 6.30 that Tuesday morning. It is a strange phenomenon, and when I told Clare about it once, she said I must have swallowed an alarm clock like the crocodile in *Peter Pan*. Mary happily does not share it, and as she was sound asleep I went for a shower and made us a cup of tea before waking her. As always we were anxious to see how Clare had spent the night, or what remained of it since we left her at 1.30 a.m., so we dressed quickly and were over in the Unit by 7.15. We found her in the middle of being washed but we were assured that the brain pressure was still fine and there had been no problems in the night. And as we were obviously in the way, we went across to the canteen for breakfast and once again succumbed to a plate of bacon and eggs washed down with tea from the Filtrona machine which I had now learnt to operate with reasonable competence.

We decided over breakfast that Mary should drive home for a short time today as she needed to get some clean things and also pop into her office. She had wanted to go home briefly the previous day but I had dissuaded her because I remembered how terrible it had been going into the empty house and seeing Clare's things. Today would be better as our 'daily' would be there, our much loved and totally indispensable Mrs Dolding, who had been coming to sort out our mess four times a week for several years. Mary had been wonderfully brave and calm through everything so far, but I knew how she would feel when she went home, and it released a lot of tension to have a good cry with another woman to comfort her.

I can best describe Clare's condition that morning by telling what happened when the neurosurgical team came in on their mid-morning ward-round. This time it was led not by Mr Sutcliffe but by his chief, Mr King, the Consultant neurosurgeon whom I now met for the first time. His acolytes were particularly deferential in the presence of the Chief himself, and I must say I too was impressed by his careful scrutiny of the charts and notes, then the very precise questions which he asked of both his entourage and the Trauma Unit staff. He reminded me very much of Mary's father, Kendal Dixon, who was Professor of Cyto-pathology at Cambridge and a fellow of my old

College, King's. He even had some of the same mannerisms, including the use of his middle rather than index finger to follow the lines of the notes as he read them. I was sorry Mary was not there to see him. He radiated calm competence and reliability, but I also had the impression, later confirmed, that he would be an engaging and genial personality when the work was done and he had a glass of decent claret in his hand.

I was relieved to see that he appeared satisfied and encouraged by Clare's progress so far. He gave her a thorough examination and produced reflexes now in all four limbs - little still on the right side but clearly discernible and improving. But best of all was when he took his ophthalmoscope and tried to look in her eyes. He was standing by her left side, and when he lifted the tightly closed and evidently still very sore lid of her swollen left eye, her left hand suddenly shot up and pushed him away so firmly that she knocked his glasses off his nose. 'Encouraging, definitely encouraging,' he said soberly as he replaced them and pretended not to have heard a smothered guffaw from one of his junior acolytes whose face had turned the colour of a beetroot. Then when I leant over from her right side where I was standing to hold her left arm down while he had another go, the most wonderful thing happened. Not only could I feel much more strength in Clare's left arm but as I held it down her right hand tried to rise. It could not do much and soon dropped back, but to see it actually moving under Clare's semi-conscious will, rather than just twitching in response to a very sharp pinch on the tender part of the upper arm, was quite wonderful.

Mr King confirmed what his Senior Registrar had said last night, that it should soon be possible to get Clare off the ventilator, for she was already proving able, and being allowed, to breathe partly by herself. I could hardly wait for Mary to come back to tell her this news. Nor were we the only Trauma Unit relatives feeling a sense of hope and relief. Len Davies in the far bed was also regaining consciousness, and when his wife Carole spoke to him he managed to open his eyes and look at her. She was so thrilled. It was still early days for both Clare and Len, but the whole Unit now seemed full of hope, and the staff reflected it as much as we did. Then suddenly we were asked to leave the Unit for a while as a new patient was being admitted. The old lady who had been in the third bed had been well enough to be transferred to one of the ordinary wards that morning.

Now the helicopter was about to land with a new accident victim, and the staff were at action stations to receive her.

After spending a few quiet minutes in the Chapel, then buying some fresh supplies of chocolate biscuits for the staff, I went back to the third floor and sat on my old friend the blue stacking chair to wait to be allowed back into the Unit. It was a very different scene now from the eerie quietness of our vigils in the middle of the night. The busy hospital at midday was like the whole world in microcosm - cosmopolitan, polyglot and infinitely varied. The dominant local immigrant group, once Jewish, is now Bangladeshi, and all the hospital signs are written in that language as well as English; but almost every race was represented among the staff, patients and visitors, all united by their common concern with healing. There can be strength as well as weakness in diversity, but only if there is a common goal which is good. Material greed, or even the natural desire for reasonable prosperity, is not enough. It needs a transcendentally good unifying aim, and as I watched this multi-ethnic hospital community working harmoniously for the common goal of healing I was reminded of a community in South Africa which had showed how the fear that motivated *apartheid* could be replaced by a unifying love which, if only the example could be cloned, could make that country one of the happiest in the world.

The community I was thinking of was the congregation of the church of St Michael and All Angels in Alexandra township near Johannesburg. Alexandra has been much in the news over recent years as one of the troubled 'black townships', but Mary and I and our then six-year-old Clare never had a moment's fear or met any unpleasantness as we used to drive from the First to the Third World many a Sunday morning simply by crossing the Louis Botha motorway which separated the 'white' suburbs from the 'non-white' in that strange society. Within a few hundred yards we were on dirt roads, driving slowly between the houses and shanties to avoid the children and chickens running about in the streets. The church itself was a very basic structure with a corrugated iron roof, but to us it represented something very beautiful.

There would usually be about a dozen white faces in the congregation, but these were only the most immediately obvious aspects of a much deeper diversity. Other countries tend to see South Africa's problems solely as a confrontation between White and Black, and - until recently at least - have naively assumed that the ANC is the voice of a united Black monolith. The guilt-complexes of Western white nations are of course understandable, and it is easier to have a simple 'good guy, bad guy' view of a situation than to wrestle with the reality of a very complex tribal society. Good guys and bad guys are not restricted to any tribal group or colour of skin, and evil though *apartheid* undoubtedly was, the conduct of the dominant Afrikaner tribe in South Africa was no worse than that of many black tribes which asserted themselves and monopolise power in almost every former colonial territory in Africa which has gained independence. Horrible as it was with its *apartheid* policies, the dominant white tribe never followed the policy of genocide against rival tribes as happened in Zimbabwe, for instance, where the Matabele army was trained by North Koreans to do some very nasty 'ethnic cleansing' of the rival Mashona lands. On the other hand even the worst excesses of the Matabele in Zimbabwe were humane compared with the example of genocidal white tribalism set by Nazi Germany, which should alone be enough to silence white supremacists. The fact is that no skin-colour has a monopoly of virtue, yet it is the unspoken assumption of white superiority which paradoxically underlies the well-intentioned naiveté of whites in comfortable Western societies who make any excuse for the evils done by blacks to other blacks while rightly castigating the oppression of blacks by whites. If I had a black skin I don't think I should want to have special allowances made for me on that score: I should prefer to be regarded as an individual, or a member of a profession, or citizen of a country. At any rate, I was glad to be regarded simply as a fellow Christian in Alexandra rather than a hated member of a dominant tribe because of the colour of my skin.

That was the great beauty of St Michael's. It was a totally mixed congregation which encapsulated what South Africa could become if the country as a whole could be motivated by the same mutual respect and unified by the same loyalty to a Higher Authority whose message to the world, perverted though it has been by man's inhumanity over the centuries, was purely one of love. As you went in, there were different piles of prayer and hymn books for the different languages. When a hymn was to be sung, one of the girls in the wonderful choir would stand up and announce the numbers in all the different books: 'Xhosa 341, Zulu 76, Tswana 124, Sotho 293, *Ancient & Modern* 92'. To hear the dear old Anglican hymnal, *Hymns Ancient & Modern*, announced among these other tribal ones gave me enormous pleasure, and the potential for strength from diversity was soon fulfilled in the joyful sound that nearly lifted the corrugated iron roof right off that church. How different from the miserable and embarrassed wheezing of the typical English congregation nowadays! We all sang our best in our different languages to the one uniting tune. It was a glorious experience and one that I miss very much.

For the leaders of communities troubled with problems of so-called race-relations, a half day spent on the blue stacking chair on the third floor of the London Hospital could be a salutary experience. It would also be nice to think that the purveyors of terrorism or violent crime might be moved by a half-day in the Trauma Unit, but I fear that individuals so evil-minded as to bomb and shoot innocent people are probably beyond redemption, at least by human means. The Unit's new patient was one of their victims. Happily she was conscious and not so badly injured that she needed ventilation, but she was in a terrible state of shock as she sat up in bed propped up with pillows and with her chest and left arm swathed in bandages. She had been blasted at point blank range by a sawn-off shotgun as she served behind the counter of a post-office. Now what sort of people are they who can do something like that to this lovely young woman in her early twenties quietly going about her daily work and harming no-one?

There is, of course, nothing new in robbery with violence or terrorism, but society does not help itself by glorifying it in so many films of appalling brutality. To glamorise the so-called 'Great' Train Robbers with a film which made them heroes to the simple-minded is surely asking for trouble and is the symptom of a sick society. Where is the documentary film of the ruined life of the coshed guard on that train and the effect on his family? That is the film which should have been made and shown on 'prime-time' television. I believe the media have a lot to answer for in their concentration on what is, to use the old-fashioned but strictly accurate word, just plain evil. As every parent knows, behaviour is largely imitative, and as long as violence is glorified, as long as terrorists have the sick satisfaction of seeing the results of their bombings on television every night and as long as youngsters on housing estates are constantly shown how others are defying the police and looting shops, we are simply propagating our problems. That is not to say there are no genuine frustrations and deprivations that need urgent attention - the horrific levels of unemployment, particularly among the young, inadequate education, the lack of moral leadership, the break-up of family life, the loss of the old conventions of decency and restraint, the availability of drugs. All the same I do believe that the visual media have a great deal more power than responsibility, and the restriction of the reporting of acts of violence and terrorism to verbal reports would, I believe, remove one of the great attractions both of hooliganism and terrorism, quite apart from the dangers of encouraging imitation.

When Mary returned she was thrilled to hear how Clare had begun to respond and had managed to knock Mr King's glasses off his nose when he tried to peer into her sore eye.

It was one of the few times I had seen Mary smile spontaneously rather than politely since before the accident. It was such a little thing, but everything is relative. Seventy-two hours ago we had thought nothing of the complex achievement of brain, nerves and hand that enabled Clare to work out and write down the solution of a quadratic equation. Now it was a triumph that she could have controlled her hand sufficiently to be able to try to push Mr King away and knock his glasses off in the process. She still looked terrible, with the top of her head bandaged, blood still seeping from the drain, the bolt sticking out of the centre of her skull, the long, pear-shaped face with its swollen eyes, neck and jaw, the wires and tubes protruding from seemingly every limb. But those limbs were becoming more responsive every hour. It was as though she was returning to us from a long, long way away. We sat one on either side of her bed, stroking her arms and legs, occasionally tickling her feet to feel if there was a response, and increasingly having to hold down her left hand as it groped for the ventilator or catheter tubes. We kept putting her beloved Leo in her left hand, and now she not only grasped him but gave him rather a rough time, waving him about then dropping him as she again groped for the prime irritant, the tube down her nose.

About 4 o'clock in the afternoon Mr Sutcliffe came in with one or two of his team, talked briefly to the nurses, examined the charts, helped himself to a chocolate biscuit, then said, 'Right then, let's get her off that ventilator.' Clare had two nurses all to herself today, Angela and a newcomer to the Unit, Michelle, who was just about to join the staff and was learning the ropes. As they got the oxygen mask ready and began to dismantle the equipment that had breathed for Clare for so long, we saw them exchange knowing looks in a mixture of disapproval and delight, which was not lost on Mr Sutcliffe.

'The anaesthetists normally do this', he explained to us, 'and make a meal of it. It takes them about two hours. My methods are cruder but quicker'. Then to our astonishment he bent over Clare's ear and said, 'Come on now, Clare, get rid of that horrible tube for us!' Her left hand groped about for a moment, then got hold of the tube and pulled it smartly out of her lungs with a sweep that would have done credit to a salmon fisherman. As the tube whirled through the air we were all spattered with flecks of phlegm, but there it was - out!

'Excellent', exclaimed Mr Sutcliffe, wiping his face with a handkerchief. 'Well done, Clare!'

'That Mr Sutcliffe!', said Angela to Michelle in an aside whose tone showed that admiration for his unconventional methods overcame professional disapproval.

For a few moments Clare coughed and spluttered as though she was drowning, but the two nurses quickly cleared her throat by the insertion of small suction tubes and placed an oxygen mask over her face. She was breathing now entirely unaided, and it was the breathing rhythms and blood-oxygen level monitors that were now critical to watch. The brain pressure monitor was still connected and exertions like these caused it to go up sharply, but even so it was within the levels of safety. As for the blood oxygen monitor, it was an amazing little thing - a tiny tube barely two inches long which fitted over her index finger and contained a light which had to be positioned over the finger nail. Heaven only knows how this monitored the level of oxygen in the bloodstream, but it did, and it became one of my jobs to try to stop Clare pushing it off with the other fingers and thumb of her left hand.

Mary and I now decided that we should begin letting friends and family know what had happened. Except for my doctor friend Hughie Webb, our Vicar and our closest business colleagues we had both been incommunicado for three days, partly for selfish and partly for altruistic reasons: we had wanted privacy for ourselves and at the same time had not wanted to upset others until we knew if Clare was likely to survive. But we could not easily put it off any longer. Mary's firm had in any case let the cat out of the bag when her brother had rung from New Zealand to ask about some problem with the tenants of his house in Cambridge, and Mary's mother would be wondering why she had not had her almost nightly phone call for so long. Mary had also found the answering machine at home totally constipated with messages, and my fax machine had run out of paper. So now that Clare was breathing by herself again and the operation had clearly been successful in reducing the brain pressure, we had the heart as well as the need to let people know. All the same, we decided to write rather than telephone, partly because we could not trust ourselves not to break down on the phone but mainly because we felt it would be less of a shock to them to read a carefully composed letter than get a call out of the blue.

The only person we wanted to ring, besides Mary's mother and brother, was our goddaughter, Frances, who is like an elder sister to Clare. Her father is an old College friend of mine who lives in South Africa, and when his daughter perplexed him by saying that she did not want to go to University but to come to England instead and try to become a silversmith, he sent her to stay with us in London. She was then seventeen, a bright, cheerful and sensible young woman with a shock of fiery red hair and the determination to face what was bound to be an uphill struggle, for apprenticeships are few and normally go to families connected with the trade. But here she was - out of Africa for the first time in her life and ready to conquer England.

For several anxious weeks she seemed to be getting nowhere, but when I visited the Training Officer of the British Jewellers' Association with whom she had corresponded before coming to London he told me not to despair. When I asked him for a candid assessment of her ability and her chances of securing an apprenticeship, he was unequivocal. 'Her portfolio is excellent', he told me. 'In fact I have seldom seen such a promising applicant in all my seventeen years in this job. She has the ability to become one of the great silver-chasers of London, which to all intents and purposes means the world. Don't worry - we'll find her something. She's too good to waste'. He was as good as his word, and just before her eighteenth birthday I had the great honour of representing her father at the indenture ceremony in the Goldsmiths' Hall, where she signed her name in a book of apprentices that went back nine hundred years.

That was nearly two years ago. Frances was no longer living with us and had her own flat nearby, but she often spent week-ends with us and came on holidays with us too. Despite the difference in their ages, she and Clare were very fond of each other, and we knew that Frances would not only want to be told but would want and be able to help. As Clare came closer to consciousness the youthful presence of her much loved 'Friend' - for the girls used to address each other as 'Friend' - would be excellent stimulation for her. But Friend's telephone at home was out of order, and as she had left the workshop when we tried there we would have to wait for the next morning to get in touch with her.

When I went to the W.H. Smith shop to buy writing paper and envelopes I decided instead to buy cards. There was a huge rack of very beautiful 'greetings cards' without pre-printed greetings, and one in particular caught my eye, for it depicted a tall and pretty girl about Clare's age wearing an Edwardian summer dress in a cornfield. It seemed to fill me with hope, and I thought it would be appropriate to carry our message of cautious optimism to our friends and relations. I bought their whole stock of that card and as we sat by Clare's bed we had quite a few to put in the hospital's post box before the last collection of the day.

It was amazing how quickly time passed. There were frequent visits from Linda the physiotherapist to keep the lungs free of phlegm, and as Clare came closer and closer to consciousness and the coughing bouts became more and more convulsive, I found myself having to hold down the right hand as well as the now powerful left as the tubes were inserted. We were now even able to joke a bit. 'You'll have to give up cigars, Clare', we'd say, and the suction tubes became 'wiggly worms' - feeble jokes, certainly, but expressing a relief of tension and a growing optimism that was shared by the staff as well as ourselves. Physiotherapists in any case are always cheerful people, full of energy and fun. At least I have never met one who wasn't. Linda certainly was, breezing in like a whiff of oxygen, quite exhilarating. She was clearly pleased at how well the fluid was coming away and confirmed her early view, that there was not much to worry about in the chest now as the ribs would mend of their own accord and the amount of fluid was decreasing nicely.

Poor Clare. After each convulsive clearance she would be exhausted and her face, which had begun to look more alive, would resume that distant look as though she was drifting away from us again deeper into unconsciousness. The reflexes would die away completely on the right arm and sometimes even the right leg at these times, and even the left hand grew feeble in its movements. It was alarming at first, but Linda told us not to worry: the monitors were all satisfactory, and gradually - each time a little more quickly - Clare's reflexes would return.

As before, we took it in turns to go for supper in the canteen, and Mary had a good talk to Carole Davies. Clare and Len were both doing well. Len was now opening his eyes quite frequently, and when Carole and Mary came back and Carole kissed him on the nose, he not only opened his eyes but gave a little smile of recognition and tried to say something. It was lovely to see Carole so happy and relieved. When she went home that night she said she was 'walking on air'. We were so happy for her and wondered if Clare might open her eyes the next day. Though the bruising was beginning to subside, her eyes were still tightly shut and so far we had seen no facial signals of recognition or expression at all except for the terrible automatic grimaces which she made when the suction tubes were pushed down her throat.

As usual we were reluctant to leave Clare and go to bed, and as usual we were bullied into it by the staff, Sarah-Jane and James that night. This time, however, we were not going back to the hostel because we had been given the little room opposite the Trauma Unit, which was now free. Though the hostel was lovely and the Superintendent most apologetic about having to move us, we were privately delighted. What did it matter that the bedroom opposite the Unit had no washing facilities? There were toilets on the landing, and the ITU Relatives' Room with its little cabinet shower in the kitchenette was nearby. No suite at the Dorchester could have been more welcome to us that night than that Spartan little room where we could sleep within twenty yards of Clare.

CHAPTER SIX

I was up early next morning, which was Wednesday, and having spent a few minutes in the Trauma Unit with Clare (and replenished the staff's supply of chocolate before the changeover) I went out and drove home before the rush-hour. Clare had had a satisfactory night, but there had been a lot of activity around Len Davies' bed and I hoped that nothing was amiss.

At that time in the morning it took me only twenty minutes to drive home, where I found Clare's budgerigar and goldfish glad to see me. The enormously fat old fish, though fed by Mrs Dolding the previous day, is used to perpetual snacks, and I found her wriggling frantically for a spoonful of her revolting dried river-shrimps. As for the bird, it was a pathetic sight. Though old, neurotic and extremely bad-tempered, she likes company and had responded to loneliness or a sense of unease by plucking a lot of her feathers out. They were all over the place, and as the wretched creature would soon be oven-ready unless she had some company, I asked our neighbours if they would look after her. Actually she had only herself to blame for being alone in the first place. She used to have a lovely, soppy husband, bigger than her but totally hen-pecked. She was sometimes so vile to him that we had to rescue him on particularly bad days and put him in a separate cage for his own protection, yet whenever we did so he would just mope in a lump of misery until he was reunited with his shrewish spouse. No husband was ever such a glutton for punishment until one day a heart-attack solved his dilemma and left his widow to face a lonely old age with no companion on which to vent her spleen.

Having collected changes of clothes and dealt with the answering and fax machines I returned to the hospital to find a happy note waiting for me in our room from Mary. 'I'm with Clare and washing her!' I popped my head round the curtains of her bed and Mary looked up with the loveliest smile on her face as she gently washed Clare's limbs. She was so happy to be doing something physical to help, and that particular smile took me straight back fourteen years: it was the smile of a mother washing her baby for the first time. But this baby gave no smiles or gurgles of delight, or even wails of discomfort. The thought that we might have a totally dependent daughter now all our lives entered my mind, and though I tried to push it away I knew at that moment what parents must feel like when the baby they have looked forward to for so long is born disabled in mind or body. I also knew how love is stronger than despair and was ready to face whatever the future might hold.

About half past ten Mr Sutcliffe came in on his morning round and said that Clare could have the head-bolt out as he was satisfied that the brain pressure no longer needed monitoring. By eleven she was being wheeled into the operating theatre for what was to be the last time, and when she returned and had been cleaned up by the nurses she looked so much better. The head-bolt and its wires were gone, as was the drain. She now had a clean, unbloodied bandage over her skull, and when Linda next came in to clear her lungs she astonished us by saying that she would be getting Clare standing up later on.

'But she is still unconscious!' I protested.

'She won't be much longer', Linda replied. 'She will be coming to quite soon, and we need to check her reflexes much more thoroughly at this stage'.

Our excitement at the prospect of Clare's early return to consciousness was tempered not only by apprehension about what consciousness would reveal but by what was happening to Len in the far bed. I had feared that something was wrong when I had seen the anxious cluster of doctors and staff round his bed earlier. Since then several doctors we had not seen before had been coming in and out, and he was linked up to even more machinery. Our hearts went out to Carole who had left him so happily only twelve hours ago. When she came in about midday it was terrible to see her poor face change when she saw and heard what was happening. Though Len's head had not been as badly damaged as Clare's, his internal bodily injuries were evidently very severe indeed, and he had now developed septicaemia which was not responding to antibiotics. His condition was deteriorating rapidly, and an hour later he was transferred to the main part of ITU, where they deal with the full range of intensive medical care rather than the trauma victims where brain damage is the main problem.

The speed of Len's reverse was terrifying. Only last night his recovery had seemed well ahead of Clare's, and I even have to confess that my joy at seeing Carole's happiness when Len had opened his eyes and recognised her with a smile had been tinged with a spot of envy. Now, as Len was wheeled away into ITU, Carole came over to us and despite her anguish was keen to ask about Clare and so pleased to hear she was doing well. Then as she was told it would be half an hour or so before she could sit with her husband in ITU, Mary took her for a coffee and they comforted each other as only two women can who share the watching and waiting over those they most love in life.

'Please God', I thought, 'don't let that happen to Clare too', and as soon as Mary returned I went down to the Chapel and prayed for Len and Clare together. 'As they have suffered together, let them recover together', I prayed, and as I said the words I knew they would. It was not self-deception or wishful thinking. It was sudden and absolute knowledge. I simply knew that neither of them would die.

By early afternoon Clare was becoming very restless. Her eyes were still tightly shut but her left hand was very active indeed, constantly trying and occasionally succeeding in getting the oxygen mask off, and when not doing that, groping for the catheter or pushing the blood-oxygen monitor off her finger. It was becoming a losing battle just to keep the mask on, and as the blood-oxygen levels were satisfactory Angela decided to take it off and just lay it upside down on her shoulder so that a stream of oxygen blew over her face. We were told to watch the monitor and if it fell below a certain level to put the mask back or at least hold it over her face for a few minutes till it went up again. Then Linda came back again, this time with one of her colleagues, and said briskly, 'Right now, Clare. Time to stand up!' She explained to us that normally the neurosurgical physiotherapists would do this - they were specialists in the rehabilitation of brain-damaged patients - but as they were short-staffed that day through illness she was going to do it herself.

It was action stations for everyone. With the ECG electrodes now disconnected and the head-bolt out there were fewer wires and tubes to worry about, but still enough with the drips, the catheter and the blood-oxygen monitor, and the oxygen mask had to be kept at the ready too. Then Linda went to the far side of the bed, took Clare under the arms and lifted her into a sitting position, kneeling on the bed behind Clare as she did so, then shuffling down the bed with her hands under Clare's shoulders while her colleague swung Clare's legs over the edge of the bed. It was a skilful performance. Linda was slightly built but amazingly strong. First she held Clare in the sitting position while her colleague tried to get her to hold up her head, and Clare did make a bit of an effort to do this though she was as helpless as a complete drunk. Then suddenly Linda made a huge effort and actually got Clare standing, bearing her dead weight by her shoulders while the colleague stood in front of Clare and looked and felt to see how much resistance there was in the hips and knees. To us it looked hopeless, but Linda was surprisingly positive. 'That's not bad', she gasped, 'not bad at all', and when she had let Clare subside again she told us she had definitely felt some resistance there, particularly on the left side, as she would expect at this stage, but not totally lacking on the right either.

The exertion also produced convulsive coughing from Clare, and as soon as she had been swung round and laid back on the bed Linda and the nurses advanced on her with the 'wiggly worms'. Poor Clare, she had no strength left even to try and push them away, but Linda seemed pleased with the amount Clare was bringing up of her own accord.

'Nothing like a bit of exercise for getting the muck up, is there, Clare?'

Clare's exhaustion for the next hour gave us chance to write to some more of our friends, then one of them to whom we had written the previous evening suddenly knocked on the door. We had told everyone not to visit or try to ring as we would keep them informed, but this particular friend would have none of that. She is devoted to Clare, and they talk to each other as sisters despite a disparity in their ages of more than half a century.

We first met Doreen about twenty years ago when she was the Chairman's secretary at the Bank for which I then worked. We saw quite a lot of each other as she lived very close to us, and I also worked closely with my Chairman from time to time. We then had our tiny cottage at Thames Ditton, the one next to Mrs Eley, and when we left England to go abroad four years later Doreen bought it from us and lives there still. And how lovely it looks under the tender care of a brilliant gardener who has had time in her retirement to turn it into a mini Sissinghurst.

Doreen is a complex character. She is a gentle person, kind, considerate and sometimes almost self-effacing in company, yet she is also tremendous fun, drives an open-topped sports car, and has that enviable knack of always looking elegant whether in her gardening clothes or dressed for Covent Garden. Clare thinks the world of her and often goes to stay. They go swimming together, visit heavy-horse farms, go to the theatre, cook, meet a variety of Doreen's friends, who include writers, potters and artists, and altogether have enormous fun. I should have known that nothing would have kept Doreen away from the hospital when she received our letter. But she was the perfect visitor. She would not come in and see Clare - she said she could not have borne it - nor would she stay above a couple of minutes. With typical sensitivity she said she had just come to give Mary and me a hug and ask if there was anything she could do to help. There was nothing of course because she had done it already, just by coming. Dear Doreen. She would not even let me go down with her to the hospital entrance. 'Just give the pretty one a hug and a kiss from me', she said, then swept into the lift with a cape flung over her shoulder and a smart beret perched at a jaunty angle on her head. She was dressed for victory, not defeat. It was just the tonic we needed.

At five o'clock our goddaughter Frances arrived. Mary had managed to catch her at her workshop, though it had been difficult to break the news gently because there was so much clattering and banging and taped music in the background. Of course she came at once, and when I met her on the landing as she came out of the lift I was a bit apprehensive about how she would react. I need not have worried. She listened carefully to what had happened, and I warned her that Clare was looking a bit grim. But her emotions were under control, and when she went in to Clare she simply sat by the bed, put her head with its tumble of glorious red hair on Clare's breast and guided her left hand over it so that she could feel it.

'Hello, Friend', she said. 'Give me a hug'. And Clare did. Though her eyes were still tightly shut, her arm was now round Frances' neck and there was clearly recognition. It was not Frances but I who lost control at that moment and left the room quickly before I disgraced myself.

When the night staff came on, they were delighted to see Clare responding so well. It was a constant battle to keep Clare from fiddling with the catheter, and she had become so adept at pushing the blood-oxygen monitor off her index-finger with her thumb and third finger that we had to lengthen the lead and transfer it to her right hand. Even so she kept managing to dislodge it from its necessary position with the light over the finger nail, for the right hand too was now becoming much more active, especially if you restrained the left, though it had not yet recovered independent movement of the individual fingers as the left had done. As for the right leg, it was nearly as responsive as the left, and when the suction tubes were inserted to clear her lungs both legs would now bend and snap to attention like a guardsman's.

Sandra and James were doing the night shift that Wednesday night, and when they came in about half past seven it was already like greeting old friends. They were so pleased to see Clare's progress but we were all worried about Len Davies, and as soon as the change-over had been completed James went across to ITU to see how he was. The news was not good. He was 'holding his own', but only with the help of constant transfusions and dialysis. Carole was expected at any time and Mary left a note for her at the ITU desk to say that they were constantly in our thoughts and prayers and that Mary would love to see her.

Though Frances was reluctant to leave Clare I insisted that she went home about ten o'clock, walked down with her onto Whitechapel Road and hailed a passing taxi. Frances protested in vain as I pressed a ten pound note into her hand. Having so nearly lost my daughter I was not going to risk my goddaughter tonight on tubes and buses and walking alone to her flat. She gave me a big hug, then I told the cabbie to take good care of her and watched her disappear down the road giving a thumb's up sign through the back window. She is a great girl. Mary and I are as proud of her as if she had been a daughter of our own. With so many youngsters going wrong it is reassuring to see a fine young woman like Frances working hard and having fun but without succumbing to the herd pressures to indulge in drugs or excessive alcohol or loose living.

We were in bed ourselves not long after midnight. Mary and Carole had had a cup of tea together, and we had met her son and daughter and their spouses. They are such a nice family. Carole also told us that Len's colleagues at work had had a 'whip round' for him and sent her over £200, which she said was very welcome as Len had always managed the finances and she had not sorted out yet where everything was. There is clearly a great camaraderie among construction workers. Len's son told me that accidents were so common on the Canary Wharf site that hardly a week went by without a collection for someone's family, and I heard more about it from Nick, who had spent six months as Accident Officer on part of that site before joining the Trauma Unit's nursing staff.

Talking one night when I was sitting up late with Clare, Nick told me that even he had been astonished by the number of accidents on that site. 'No-one needed telling to wear his hard hat there', he said. 'They were terrified'. Then he explained to me that Canary Wharf was using the so-called 'fast track' method of construction, which involved having different phases of the work which are normally done sequentially done simultaneously instead. He said it was chaos, with so many different trades and sub-contractors and sub-contractors of sub-contractors all trying to work on the same building at the same time that half of the men scarcely seemed to know who they were working for. In Nick's view safety was being sacrificed for speed, and certainly there were a lot of bloody victims on the altar of commercial greed, for the accident figures were staggering. He told me stories of men so afraid of losing their wages that one had actually pleaded with him to strap up a broken arm so that he could get back on the job. Perhaps it was only justice that Canary Wharf has proved a commercial disaster for its hybristic developers. A less grandiose and more humane scheme might have been - and would certainly deserve to have been - more successful.

CHAPTER SEVEN

This morning, Thursday, I again drove home very early. The answering machine was again jammed with messages from friends who had learnt of Clare's accident, and I could hardly open the front door for the little heap of cards behind it. There were also messages from many of our neighbours asking if they could do anything to help, and as I looked out of the window I could see that some kind person had watered the garden and mown the lawn. I was very touched by their kindness.

My fax machine too had been busy, and among the messages were two which I shall always keep. They were from two of our dearest friends, Philip and Denyse Bulmer. Phil was at College with me and was my Best Man when Mary and I were married twenty-four years ago. The following year he married Denyse, and when their first child was born the year after that - long before we had Clare - we became her godparents.

That was Sally, who is now a very beautiful, sensible and delightful young woman of twenty-three. But Phil and Denyse faced tragedy with two other children. Their second, Louise, was severely spastic, and their third, Mary, died only a few hours after she was born. Happily the doctors advised that there was no genetic reason at all why future children should not be perfectly normal, and subsequently they had another daughter, Caroline, who is Clare's age, and - something of an accident, but a happy one - a little boy, Jack, born when Denyse was forty-five. Both Caroline and Jack are strong, healthy children, and thank God they are, because their parents had been through so much with Louise.

No parents could have done more for a disabled child than Phil and Denyse had done. When she was still a baby they had investigated every possible treatment both in England and abroad, and having discovered that there was a centre in Philadelphia which had apparently produced remarkable improvements in severely spastic children, he had not hesitated to borrow money from his employers and take Louise out to America. The treatment, known as 'patterning', involved constant manipulation of the child for many hours a day to try to imprint on a new and undamaged part of the brain the basic crawling movements which develop instinctively in the normal baby. The theory was that the potential for subsequent development could be latent in undamaged parts of the brain but unable to be released until the earlier stages of a child's natural programme had been completed. In other words, if the crawling stage, which is normally instinctive, could be taught by repetitive movement, this could stimulate future stages of natural physical development once the gap in the sequence had been artificially bridged.

When Phil returned he had been very impressed by what he had seen, and although Louise had been assessed as very severely impaired, they were determined to try the treatment. They converted their large living room into a virtual gymnasium, with exercise tables, graded slopes so that the crawling could be assisted by gravity, and devices to take some of the weight off her body by suspension. They advertised among local church and community groups for helpers in the programme, and soon there were teams of volunteers helping Louise with the very intensive, repetitive programme of exercise prescribed by the Philadelphia institute. Little Sally was marvellous too. Phil and Denyse were admittedly careful not to starve her of attention, but even so it says much for the niceness of her nature that she never resented the concentration on Louise and was always kind to her handicapped little sister.

For a time it all seemed very worthwhile. When Phil took Louise back to America two months later for another assessment, she had improved substantially and he came back full of optimism. Efforts were redoubled, and a hard core of dedicated helpers gave unstintingly of their time to continue the programme. Sadly, however, the progress did not continue, and after several more weeks Phil and Denyse had to admit that there was no point in carrying on at that level of intensity, which was also hard on the child as well as her helpers. Having done all they could to stimulate physical development, they would now concentrate on intellectual development while finding or making the best mechanical aids to make her as mobile and comfortable as possible.

We were living abroad at that time, but whenever we visited England and stayed a few days with these dear friends, we found Louise with some wonderful new devices, often designed by Phil himself. She was going to a school for handicapped children, and when she was at home her parents did everything possible to stimulate her. She could not speak at all, and her hands had almost no control. She could, however, move her head, and soon Phil had designed her an electric wheel-chair which she could operate by pressing her chin on three large pressure-switches. I remember taking her for a trial run on a disused race-track, Louise squealing with delight as she put herself suddenly in reverse and we had to charge after her to stop her falling out. She also managed to learn simple reading. You could hold up a card with the word 'window', for example, and she would look at the window. Similarly she could choose what she wanted to eat or drink by making an enthusiastic noise when shown the card with the name of the item she wanted. It was not as if the child lacked intelligence, and that in a way only intensified the tragedy. You could see the frustration in her eyes as she longed to join in conversation, and sometimes she would burst out laughing at a joke even before anyone else had got it.

As she grew older, the difficulties increased, not least because she became too heavy for Denyse to handle without help, for Denyse is very petite and Louise grew taller then her mother. Then three years ago her spine was curving so badly that her doctors recommended an operation to insert a metal rod into her back to keep her upright. To have to decide on so painful and serious an operation for oneself is bad enough, but to do it for a loved one who could not really understand must have been terrible. Poor Louise went almost to skin and bone afterwards and must have had a lot of pain, but it had to be done and was happily a great success. When we last saw Louise it was her twenty-first birthday and she was looking happy, cheerful and very pretty in a gorgeous party-dress.

Louise is fortunate in that her parents have been totally committed to helping her make the best of her limited potential. They have not only given unstintingly of themselves and their own time and energy and love but have battled against obstinate, rule-bound local authorities to get grants for her and place her in the best possible environment. Of course there are many claims on local authority funds and there have to be regulations, but some of the bureaucratic absurdities against which they had to fight were mindless. Moreover there is little provision for that difficult period when a child is over sixteen and still needing schooling beyond the basic school-leaving age. The fact that she has such severe physical handicaps means that a young woman like Louise needs more, not less, education. She needs continuing intellectual stimulation in an educational environment: she cannot suddenly be transferred to a home for adults to sit in a chair all day nor can her parents be expected to cope at her own home on a full-time basis, even though her father has built her her own ground-floor suite in the garden and equipped it with all available aids for the handicapped. There needs to be more provision for higher education for the disabled too, for this is an area which is severely lacking at present.

The home where Louise now lives, and which has mercifully just been reprieved from the threat of closure, is outstanding. It has a wide range of degrees of disability among its residents, some as badly handicapped as Louise, being incapable of speech or of controlling their limbs, others able to walk and talk but needing a sheltered and educational environment. All the residents are young adults and the staff treat them as such, not as big babies. The atmosphere is so healthy and natural. Any initial feeling of embarrassment soon disappears when you get among these young people, and though it is hard to understand what some of them say, you have to learn to be as patient with them as they are being with you, and when you become attuned to a speech defect you can be very surprised at the quality of thought that is being expressed. Not that you should be. That terribly handicapped scientific genius Professor Hawking, author of the all-time best-seller *A Brief History of Time,* is formidable proof that having something wrong with the communication system need not mean that there is anything wrong with the intellect.

Mary and I had not visited Louise in this home until the day of her unforgettable twenty-first birthday party. Phil and Denyse had arranged a surprise. The staff, enthusiastic conspirators in the plot, had helped Louise to organise a party for her friends, with a disco and some eats and drinks. Then as the party was under way, up rolled a motor coach with her parents and about forty family friends, including ourselves, all in fancy dress. People had gone to enormous trouble. There were Dickensian characters, Marco Polo, TV characters, a Sherwood Forest contingent of Robin Hood, Friar Tuck and Maid Marion, Sir Frances Drake, several clowns, a splendid tramp and, most hilarious of all, Phil himself as a pantomime dame. Denyse confessed to me later that she had feared that the excitement might be too much for Louise and send her into spasm, but she need not have worried. The cry which Louise gave was one of pure delight when that improbable crowd of party-goers all came in and began crocodiling round her, dispensing presents and giving her a birthday kiss. I certainly have never enjoyed a party more. It would be criminal to close a home like this for want of funds, but Government and local authority cuts are bedevilled by that absurd cliché 'across the board', which is surely the last thing one wants. Cost-cutting should be prioritised and highly selective, not an equal slice out of everything. And a home like Louise's should be sacrosanct in any civilised society.

Having been through so much themselves with Louise, the Bulmers understood better than anyone what we were going through now with Clare, and as Phil had not been able to get me on the phone, he had sent me two faxes - one the previous day, when they had received my card, and a second this morning. This is what he wrote, addressed not just to Mary and me but to Clare too.

'Dear Peter, Mary and Clare,

We were so shocked and so saddened to hear from you this morning about Clare's accident. We hope and pray that things have improved since then.

We have a very powerful prayer chain at St Paul's in Camberley and we have put Clare on it this morning.

We know what trauma and heartache you must be going through at this difficult time... but look outside, it is a beautiful spring day, a time for growth and rebirth. We hope and pray that Clare will make a full and speedy recovery.

With all our love,
Phil and Denyse.'

I had never heard of a prayer chain before and I was very touched to think that a large number of people in Camberley, where the Bulmers live, were taking it in turns day and night to maintain a perpetual outpouring of prayer for a named list of those who in the words of the old prayer-book are 'in sorrow, need, suffering or any other adversity'. Some they know personally but others not, and it was rather wonderful to think of prayers for Clare emanating in a constant cycle from the human equivalent of a Tibetan prayer-wheel.

The healing power of prayer seems to me not a simple matter but highly complex. Christ himself could heal by touch or word, but the uncertainties and failures even of the disciples themselves should warn us against the naiveté of looking for instant cures by layings-on of hands. Recent sessions in London by American tele-evangelists have been both crude and cruel. One answer to generations of prayer for healing has come in the skills and dedication of doctors, scientists and technicians and the existence of a health service available to all. Another comes in the strength that you yourself feel just from knowing that you or your loved ones are being prayed for. But there is a third, which concentrates love directly as a healing power on the recipient. I believe that the power of love can be willed into a patient by the loved ones' thoughts and prayers even if the patient is unconscious. We speak of those who have given up the struggle and those who fight, sometimes with miraculous results as will-power occasionally seems able to frustrate the ravages of the most appalling and usually deadly diseases. And whether it does so purely spiritually, or physically by stimulating the body's own defence-systems, may be a false distinction. It may be both. Indeed, the spirit may well be as material as other, if clumsier, invisible influences such as radio waves. Christianity, after all, is a materialist faith, proclaiming the resurrection of the body, and this has never seemed to me to require the physical resurrection of an individual, physical body in the same state as it was just before death, like that of Lazarus. It would be no less 'physical' and much more 'real' in the philosophical sense for components of individual personality to be preserved in some material form which, like radio waves, is unapproachable by the five unaided senses.

It is at times like this that you really discover the quality of friendship. Phil's second letter, written and faxed over to me just a few minutes before I arrived at the house, speaks for itself:

'Dear Peter, Mary and Clare,

You have all been constantly in our thoughts and prayers since we heard of Clare's accident. We have done very little work and had very little sleep since then.

We feel that we can best help by meeting with you as soon as possible. We could come to London at any time and at short notice.

Alternatively if you feel you can get away for a few hours and would benefit from a walk in the countryside with some friends, please come and see us here.

Please let us know how you are. We hope and pray that the news will be better than your letter.

With all our love,
Phil and Denyse'.

I rang Phil and Denyse at once. I had not realised that my letter to them on the cornfield card had been so shocking. I had deliberately written only after Clare seemed to be out of danger and I had tried to sound as hopeful as possible, but I had clearly not fooled my old friends. It was good to talk to them, to tell them what had happened and how Clare was now off ventilation, was gradually coming round and was showing signs of responses on both sides of her body. They asked if they should come at once, but I persuaded them to leave it till the weekend when Clare would perhaps be awake and able to recognise them. I tried to keep the emotion out of my voice but Phil obviously knew so well what we were going through that I eventually choked and promised to ring again in the evening. When I had pulled myself together I quickly rang one or two other friends, including of course Hughie Webb and our Vicar in Lancashire. They were glad to hear of Clare's progress, though it was early days, and as I spoke to them I began to feel as hopeful as I was trying to sound. And though I was still haunted by seeing the sudden relapse of Len Davies, I was not prepared for the shock which awaited for me when I returned to the hospital.

It was about 9.30 in the morning when I got back. Clare had now been moved to the bed by the window on the other side of the room which the Post Office girl had been in: her injuries had happily turned out to be less serious than had been feared and she had been transferred to an ordinary ward. When Clare eventually opened her eyes it would be pleasanter to be by the window, from which she would be able to see the helicopter taking off and landing on the rooftop helipad. The staff also liked to keep new or ventilated patients on the one side, and those who had come off ventilation on the other. There was a new patient too, opposite Clare in the place where Len Davies had been. This was the Managing Director of a big company who had missed decapitation by inches when he had been struck by the rotor of his helicopter as he visited one of his factories. As it was, he had taken a chunk out of the back of his head, but mercifully it was less serious that it looked and he was already off ventilation. A little cluster of smartly dressed executives were fussing around him rather foolishly, some possibly assessing their chances in the promotion stakes if the Chief was incapacitated for long. But the staff soon got rid of them so that he could get some rest.

The curtains were drawn round Clare's bed when I came in but I assumed she was just being washed and did not realise anything was wrong until I popped my head through to tell Mary I was back. One look at her face was enough to tell me. Moira and Michelle were on duty that morning with Steve, the senior nurse in the Unit, and Moira had just taken a blood sample from Clare. 'She is a bit flat this morning,' said Moira, and Mary added quietly, 'She has got an infection of some sort'. My heart sank. 'O God, no,' I thought, 'not like poor Len'.

One of the neurosurgeons then came in with a lady physician and did some reflex-testing. I could tell from the glances they exchanged that they were seriously worried. 'We are taking blood tests immediately', the doctor explained, 'to find out what it is. Try not to worry. We are giving antibiotics already, and when we have the test results we can target any specific problem'.

Moira gave several injections through the various taps in Clare's arm and leg, then we sat by her bed, kissed her face and stroked her limbs. But the response was feeble. Her face was puffy, her neck and jaws more swollen, and she looked to be drifting away from us again. Mary then told me that Len had deteriorated badly in the night and poor Carole had had a private interview with the Consultant, who had warned her that he now had less than a 50/50 chance of pulling through. His whole system, including his kidneys, was packing up, and though they were taking biopsies they could not get at the root of the infection nor find antibiotics that seemed able to counter it.

I left Mary and Clare for a few minutes and went down to the Chapel. Mercifully it was empty because I am afraid I broke down completely. Then I prayed with all my heart for Clare and Len together, and again I felt the certainty that they would both survive. I felt it so strongly that I felt ashamed of doubting it. I then wrote a note to the Chaplain to tell him about Len and ask him to visit Carole in ITU. There was a little box on the wall for requests for prayers or visits which was opened every two hours. I did not know what denomination Carole was, but it did not seem to matter. She needed some comfort, and the Chaplain was such a patently good man that I knew she would not reject his approach.

That morning was one of the longest I ever remember, though they waste no time in the Trauma Unit. The blood test results were back in less than an hour, whereupon Moira called the physician, who came at once. Mary and I could see the relief on their faces as they read the report. 'It seems to be nothing sinister', said the doctor reassuringly. 'Clare has a low-grade infection which should quickly respond to what we are giving her already. It is not uncommon at this stage. The labs are doing blood-cultures to identify the specific organism in case we have problems. That will take forty-eight hours, but don't worry. The preliminary analysis indicates that we're not dealing with anything too nasty'. By midday we could see for ourselves that Clare was reviving. Though still giving no facial expressions or opening her eyes, she was once again physically active, first only on the left side, then on both, and soon she was keeping us busy stopping her getting at the catheter or pulling at the oxygen mask which lay beside her on the pillow or pushing the blood-oxygen level monitor off the finger of her right hand.

Injections and close monitoring continued, but Clare was soon able to dispense with oxygen altogether, though it was kept in readiness in case of need. Mr Sutcliffe came in about midday and was happy to see Clare responding so well to the antibiotic. The rate of change, whether of deterioration or improvement, can be astonishingly rapid. Further blood samples were taken and analysed, and within a matter of two or three hours all evidence of infection had gone and the blood was clear again.

I began now to realise the importance of the unseen army of laboratory staff who back up the front-line troops on the wards. The number of biochemical tests performed each day in a major hospital on blood, urine, sputum and other bodily fluids and tissues runs into many hundreds, and while they vary greatly in difficulty and urgency, all require meticulous precision not only in carrying them out but in the recording and transmission of the results, for a careless labelling or categorisation of urgency could be fatal to a critically ill patient.

About 2.30 Linda appeared with a wheel-chair and said it was high time we got Clare up. We could hardly believe our ears, but Linda cheerfully brought the chair round to the side of the bed and in no time at all Moira and Michelle were easing the groggy child into it while Mary held the catheter and I sorted out the drip.

'Come on now, Clare, sit up!' ordered Linda, and she kept making Clare lift her drooping head.

Then Steve came over and said, 'You know, Moira, it's a lovely day and I'm sure Clare would enjoy a breath of fresh air in the garden. I can manage here, now we are left with only one other patient'.

'Are you quite sure?', said Moira, and Michelle loyally suggested that she could stay, but Steve was adamant. 'No, you must both go with Clare', he insisted. 'It's so unusual for us to have only two patients in here and neither on ventilation, so make the most of it and take Clare outside. It's a glorious day'.

It was indeed a glorious day, in every way. I asked if I could propel the chair myself - I thought I should get used to it as soon as possible - and off we set with Mary on one side keeping Clare upright and managing the lift buttons and so on, Michelle on the left with the drip which was keeping Clare nourished and hydrated intravenously, and Moira bringing up the rear with a portable oxygen and resuscitation kit 'just in case'.

Out onto the landing we went, into the lift, down to the ground floor, through the rear of the front part of the hospital, past the cancer and radiotherapy centre and out into the central courtyard, where one or two little groups of staff and visitors were sitting on the forms enjoying the beautiful air. It was the most perfect spring day, more like May than April but prevented from being uncomfortably hot by a refreshing little breeze, heavily scented with blossom. We stationed ourselves by a bench under the shade of a mulberry tree and kept talking to Clare and encouraging her to open her eyes and look at the world again.

We had not been out for many minutes when a familiar white-coated figure hailed us and came across the lawn. 'Hello, Clare', he said cheerfully, 'it's nice to see you up and about'. It was Dr Geoff Tothill, senior houseman in the neurosurgical team, and a most delightful man. He had just been out to buy a bag of tangerines from a stall on Whitechapel Road, and taking out four of them he began to juggle them most expertly. It was just the stimulation Clare needed.

'Look, Clare, look at Dr Geoff juggling with the tangerines!' we all cried, and she did, opening her eyes for the first time in five days. As the tangerines whirled through the air, giving off the most delicious smell, Clare was doing her best to keep her eyes open, though one was still very swollen and the brightness of the light even under the mulberry tree must have hurt them. Then we all clustered round her chair. 'Look, Clare, it's Mummy and Daddy, and this is Dr Geoff, and these are two new friends, Moira and Michelle. It's lovely to have you back with us, Clare'.

Clare did not move her head from side to side but she clearly focused on each of us in turn, though there was no facial expression at all or any attempt to speak, just the occasional bout of coughing. She also tired quickly and could not keep her eyes open for long, but even so she was clearly interested in what was going on around her and appeared to be listening intently. It was another breakthrough, and the two nurses and the young surgeon were as delighted as we were. All the same, as I looked at those two lovely young women holding down highly skilled and worthwhile jobs - then at poor Clare who so short a time ago had been so full of energy and life, with all her faculties intact and seemingly unlimited opportunities before her - I wondered again if she would ever be like Moira and Michelle, or stay in a wheel-chair all her life, or end up somewhere in between.

Geoff was a delightful character too, and obviously as great a favourite with the staff as with the patients. He was highly intelligent and skilled but also full of fun, totally unstuffy and - as was clear from the reaction of the girls - extremely handsome. He amused us by describing himself as a professional juggler who moonlighted as a brain-surgeon. Apparently he and a friend had found a juggling shop one day near London Bridge, and being unable to resist going in to an establishment rejoicing in the name 'Balls Up', they had both bought a juggling set and had an hour's lesson, after which, if you cannot keep three balls in the air, you get your money back. Now he had evidently become quite expert and told us it was not only fun for parties and for amusing patients, especially the children, but also aided dexterity generally and was curiously relaxing. We also discovered that he was in the Air Force Reserve and loved parachuting. Moira reminded him that he had promised to take her sky-diving, and I could not help thinking that Geoff and Moira would make an extraordinarily handsome couple. But I gathered later that he was engaged to someone else.

We stayed out about half an hour after Geoff had gone, but Clare did not open her eyes again, and as she seemed to be very tired we took her back. Even by hospital standards she must have looked quite a sight with her bandaged head flopping on her chest and an entourage of nurses holding drips and resuscitation kits. People could not help looking, but then turned away as you caught their eye. English folk are so reserved and afraid of giving offence that they can rarely react naturally and easily to the disabled. I had myself never known whether to look away, to avoid embarrassing the handicapped person and his relatives, or to look straight at him, which could appear rude. After all, to force yourself to act naturally is a paradox and can't be done. At any rate I was now on the receiving end of a variety of stares, surreptitious glances and embarrassed aversions of the eye as we trundled Clare back to the Trauma Unit, though curiously enough I felt no embarrassment myself at all. As the Chaplain had said, 'You must be proud of her *now'*, and I was.

CHAPTER EIGHT

Clare had been exhausted by her trip to the garden, particularly as the movement had loosened the fluid from her lungs and Linda had given her a volcanic session of lung-clearing as soon as she was back in bed. She was very quiet for about two hours, but when Frances came in the evening she perked up again and opened her eyes to look at her - still however without speaking or smiling but quite active with her limbs. Leo and her teddy bear were having a rough time of it, as was Frances herself when she put her head on Clare's breast and Clare gave her a very tight hug indeed.

It was such a relief to see Clare still so responsive after our scare in the morning, but though I felt terribly tired after seeing Frances to a taxi about 10.30, I could not sleep that night. I was still haunted by having seen the speed at which infections could take hold, and while Clare's seemed to have been brought quickly under control, the news about Len Davies was no better. I got up twice in the night to check that Clare was still all right and had tea and biscuits and a good chat with the night staff, Sarah-Jane and James.

Friday dawned another beautiful day, and after an early shower I had a good walk in the clear morning air and felt much refreshed. I rang Mary's brother in New Zealand, twelve hours ahead of us, and was able to give him the good news about Clare's progress. How extraordinary it seemed to be sitting in a car in a London street at 6.30 in the morning and able to dial direct from a car-phone to the other side of the world where they were sitting down to supper. The line was absolutely clear, clearer in fact than on many a local call.

As Mary was still asleep I did not disturb her but left her a little note and went for breakfast in the canteen. She was still asleep when I returned, so I woke her gently with a cup of tea and the news that Clare had had a good night and there was no recurrence of the infection. As a new patient was being admitted, it was some time before we could go and sit with Clare, but Mr Sutcliffe saw us in the corridor and took us on one side to speak to us.

'I need to talk to you about what could happen now that Clare is waking up', he began. 'We are very encouraged by her progress so far, and I have arranged for her to go for a detailed assessment by the neurosurgical physiotherapists in their gym this afternoon. We may then transfer her onto one of the wards, either the Neurosurgical Ward or the Children's. We haven't decided yet. In size she is an adult, but there are some fairly upsetting sights in the main Neurosurgical Ward and it may be better if we can get her into one of the Paediatric Wards, which are in Garden House, the classical-looking building on the other side of the courtyard where I hear you took Clare yesterday. Vicky is there too, so it's not all little ones. I've also arranged, by the way, for Clare and Vicky to have their sessions in the gym together this afternoon: it will all help to stimulate Clare'.

This was typically thoughtful and we said how grateful we were. Mary's only concern was whether or not she could continue to sleep at the hospital, but Mr Sutcliffe assured her that there was a whole suite of rooms for parents needing to stay with their children on the first floor of Garden House and we should certainly be allotted one. He did, however, want to warn us about the possible problems we might face. 'As Clare regains full consciousness', he explained, 'you may have to cope with psychological as well as physical problems. Brain injury patients commonly become extremely irritable, sometimes abusive and occasionally violent. It doesn't always happen but it is not uncommon and you must be prepared for it. I don't want to alarm you unnecessarily, but you could find that your daughter has a different personality from the one you were used to'.

'Is it usually a passing phase or can it be permanent?' I asked.

'It can be permanent', he replied, 'but it is much more often a passing phase, though it can last quite a long time. It would not be surprising really when you consider all she has been through. On the other hand it may not happen at all. Vicky, for example, showed no obvious changes of mood or temperament, and let's hope that that will be the case with Clare too. There are also certain physical barriers for Clare to cross, the main one being the ability to swallow without choking. Until now she has been fed entirely intravenously. Today we must see if she can take food by mouth'.

Back in the Trauma Unit we saw a fearfully injured young man in Clare's old bed, his body almost covered with iodine and with the full resuscitation machinery attached. He was on the same close monitoring programme which Clare had had at first, and I wondered how on earth these nurses stand the constant emotional as well as mental and physical strain of this most exacting work, which really is a matter of life and death. Sandra was on duty with Moira and

Michelle, and she gave us a pile of cards which had come for Clare. There was also a most beautiful bunch of pink roses from Clare's godparents in Yorkshire, our dear friends Peter and Annette Howdle. They have no children of their own and are Clare's guardians if anything were to happen to Mary and me. I have always felt comforted to think that Clare would be taken into such a good home if we were to die, and had never considered the possibility that Clare might die first. The Howdles were terribly upset when they received my letter, but I had a long talk with them on the phone and persuaded them not to come down yet.

An intriguing square box had also been delivered, and when we opened it - with Clare watching intently but expressionless - three jolly gas balloons soared out tethered by strings and depicting the cartoon character Garfield the Cat in medical mode. It was a lovely gift, and when we looked to see who it was from I was not surprised to see the names of Ivana and Simon, my former secretary and her husband. Ivana had been my secretary for eight years, ever since we had returned from overseas, and had loyally followed me through three changes of job. She was the perfect secretary - not only supremely efficient in all the secretarial skills of shorthand, word-processing and administration but totally unflappable, calm in crises, able to deal disarmingly with the most difficult people and blessed with a delightful sense of humour. Clare was very fond of her, and nothing could have been more typical of Ivana's thoughtfulness than this box of gaily coloured balloons that waved about cheerfully and provided exactly the sort of stimulation Clare needed.

Clare was keeping her eyes open a lot of the time now, and was forever pulling at her drip and catheter tube. The oxygen mask had been abandoned completely by now as her blood-oxygen levels were well up and she was breathing strongly and normally. The Captain of Industry in the bed opposite and his charming wife were so pleased to see Clare more alert, and when suddenly the emergency helicopter took off with a roar from its roof-top pad, he called to her to look at it and she did so, following it carefully with her eyes and seeming to understand what it was. But there was something eerie about the intensity of Clare's silent and expressionless watching, and nothing we could do would induce her to try to speak.

Fresh stimulation arrived with a knock on the door. It was two of Clare's school-friends, Alice and Charlie (really Charlotte). I went out to see them and was unthinkingly about to bring them in when Michelle suggested I kept them outside till they had tidied Clare up a bit. Having got used to her appearance and seen such improvement myself, I had forgotten quite how shocking she would still look to a couple of fifteen-year-olds standing bravely in the corridor clutching their little presents. I therefore took them into our room for a few minutes and tried to prepare them. I explained that Clare could not yet speak and had had a serious operation on her head but that I thought she would love to see them if they did not feel it would upset them too much. I reassured them - and hoped it was true - that Clare was recovering rapidly and there was nothing to worry about. I also told them that Clare would not be disfigured in any way, for though she had a big operation scar right across her forehead, it was behind her hair line and would not be visible when her hair grew again.

In a few minutes Mary came in to say that they had got Clare up and put her in the wheel-chair so that we could all go to the garden. That was an excellent idea of Moira's because the young man in Clare's old bed was in a terrible state, and it would in any case be much nicer for the girls to see Clare outside in more normal conditions. So off we trundled again, myself pushing the chair and Mary watching the drip (the catheter looking after itself, being clipped to the side of the chair out of sight under Clare's rug). Michelle had tied a silk scarf round Clare's forehead so that the scar did not show, and with her hair having been washed and blow-dried that morning she did not look too bad, despite the icon-like face curiously elongated by the swollen neck and jaw and one eye still quite discoloured with bruises.

The central courtyard where we had sat the previous afternoon under the mulberry tree on Clare's first outing was now full of contractors' machinery, but Moira took us round to another little garden at the side of Garden House, which housed the paediatric wards. We parked Clare's chair on the lawn and Charlie and Alice sat on the grass on either side of her. They were great. They chatted away to her about school, the foibles of various teachers, the antics of class-mates and what they were going to do in the Easter holidays to come. Again, Clare listened intently and seemed to understand, but we still waited in vain for any attempt to speak or answer a question.

After half an hour we thought the girls had probably had enough so we took Clare back, but they had done very well and their parents could be proud of them. Some fifteen-year-olds would have clammed up in embarrassment and others would not have dared to come in the first place, but Alice and Charlie were made of sterner stuff. They were also, like Clare, keen supporters of Tottenham Hotspurs Football Club with Garry Lineker as their common hero, and I think it was more than my imagination that Clare seemed particularly attentive when his latest exploits came into their conversation. Mary and I thanked them most sincerely for coming, and they went off cheerfully, promising to come again. They left lovely little gifts for Clare together with a huge 'get well' card signed by all the girls in her class, which now joined the others on an already crowded window sill.

'I think it's time we tried Clare on some food by mouth', said Moira when we were back in the Unit. 'She needs something tasty and semi-solid, a mousse or a custard to start with'.

I went at once to W.H. Smith's on the ground floor and selected from their fridge two little pots of chocolate mousse and one of custard. I also bought a couple of small boxed drinks with straws, one of Ribena and one of fresh orange juice. Then I hurried back.

'This is very important', explained Moira. 'Clare needs to come off the drip but the way she pulls at everything means that she would never tolerate a tube into her stomach down her nose, which is the only other way of feeding her. So let's see what she can do. The trip in the fresh air should have given her an appetite'.

I showed Clare the chocolate mousse, opened it and put a little on a plastic teaspoon.

'Touch her lips with it for a start', advised Sandra, who had come over to watch, and when I did so, out came a little pink tongue, licked it off and swallowed. You could have heard a pin drop, the tension was so great.

'Would you like a bit more?' I asked. Clare opened her mouth at once, took a half-spoonful of the mousse and again swallowed perfectly.

'Thank God for that!' exclaimed Sandra, with almost tangible relief. 'That is one of the biggest hurdles overcome'. And when Clare went into the paediatric ward and I saw some other brain-damaged children I would fully understand why. In the meantime Clare was licking her lips for more, and after a couple more spoonfuls of the mousse we tried the Ribena drink through a straw.

'Gently does it, Clare', said Mary, and the nurses stood prepared to deal with a choking fit if it went down the wrong way. But there was no problem at all. Clare sucked and swallowed perfectly, then polished off the rest of the chocolate mousse. I had often thought those little pots of mousse and tiny boxed drinks outrageously expensive, but these two were beyond price, and to this day I never see them on the refrigerated shelves of a shop or petrol station without remembering that marvellous moment when Clare ate and drank for the first time.

We put Clare back to bed now as she was clearly tired by the effort and excitement of the morning, but how much better she looked with the drip out. The catheter was the only tube left in now, though there were still taps on her limbs through which injections could be given, blood taken or tubes reconnected in case of need. The nasty-looking tap in her neck, however, was removed, as it could be a source of infection. Then Mr Sutcliffe and Dr Britto came in to see her, and when they heard that she had eaten and drunk without difficulty they were clearly delighted and very relieved. A smile appeared even on the saturnine countenance of the cautious Senior Registrar. As for young Dr Britto, he looked as though he would have raised a cheer if his chief had not been there.

'Right then', said Mr Sutcliffe, 'you're due at the neurosurgical gym at 3.30 sharp, Clare, and then, if the physios are happy, you can go straight to a ward in Garden House rather than coming back here. What do you say to that, eh?' No response. 'Well never mind. You're doing well even if you won't talk to us yet. The great thing is you are swallowing naturally. There's plenty of time'.

We packed up all Clare's things and put them with our own in our room to collect later. I then telephoned to Hughie Webb with the good news about Clare's eating and drinking, and his response was so ecstatic that I realised more than ever how critical this step had been. Mary went to see if Carole Davies was in ITU, to find out if Len was doing any better and to let her know that Clare was going over to Garden House, but not finding her there she left her a little note. At 3 o'clock Mary helped the nurses to dress Clare in jeans and a T-shirt, then at quarter past we set off under Moira's guidance to the neuro-gym in the Outpatients' Wing. It was an emotional moment to see Clare dressed again and leaving the Trauma Unit for the last time, even though it was in a wheel-chair.

Moira explained that there was a subterranean way of getting to the gym without going outside if it was raining, but on a lovely day like this she would take us overland. So out we went into the courtyard, past Garden House and out into the street at the back of the hospital, but instead of going straight along the main street and into the main entrance of the Outpatient Building she took us up a side street which led to the main Accident and Emergency entrance, where Clare had been admitted from the Westminster only six days ago. It seemed like six years. Then just before we got to the ambulance drop, she cut through a gate in the wall on our left, through a door with heavy strips of plastic draught-excluders - Clare's left hand helping feebly to push them aside - and down a long corridor to what she called the Torture Chamber.

Moira introduced us to Ros Wade, the Senior Physiotherapist, but anyone less like a torturer would be hard to imagine. She was a very beautiful young woman, and as cheerful and attractive in personality as in appearance. The gym over which she presided was a large, high room, with two beds at each end. There was a big cupboard full of equipment, a small dais with a flight of four steps at either side for practising stair-climbing, parallel bars at waist height for walking practice, and lots of gymnastic and medicine balls of all colours and diameters, including one - my favourite - which was over a yard across and pillar-box red. There was also a table and chairs and a sink with tea-making equipment, which was immediately pressed into service to make a pot of tea for Mary and me and for a patient who had just finished his session.

This was a man in his forties called Nigel, who told me he had picked up a virus in America which had clearly played havoc with his nervous system. His poor hands were twisted at a strange angle, and he could not control his fingers sufficiently to hold a cup. He held his mug between the lower parts of his palms, and by leaning over could just manage to tip it sufficiently to drink, but it was safer to use a straw. He had clearly been through a terrible time, but he was a cheerful soul with a ready wit and formidable power of repartee. We enjoyed several good chats and jokes in the days that followed.

While I helped Nigel to some tea, Ros and one of her assistants, another Michelle, wheeled Clare over to one of the beds at the far end of the gym. Putting aside the chair's foot-plates they deftly lifted her up and swung her round into a sitting position on the edge of the bed, Michelle moving quickly to the far side of the bed from where she could put her hands under Clare's shoulders to take the weight and keep her from slumping over while Ros proceeded to examine Clare from the front.

'Come on, Clare, keep your head up!' said Ros briskly. 'Look at me! That's right.' For a moment Clare managed to hold her head up, then she was swung round and laid on her back on the bed for Ros to do a full examination of all her reflexes. She tested reflexes in the legs and feet by supporting the bent leg under the knee and tapping the front of the leg just below the knee with an instrument called a patellar hammer, which had a disc at the end of its shaft. She then took each limb in turn, manipulated it and asked Clare to push against her in various positions, from which she got a determined if feeble response. I was keen to go over and watch more closely, but I felt it would be rude to Nigel, who was in the middle of an amusing story. In the meantime a porter came in wheeling Vicky in her chair and took Nigel back to his ward.

I had of course seen Vicky the previous Sunday when her parents brought her into the Trauma Unit, but I was anxious to talk to her and see how well she spoke. Though rather shy - which I gathered she had always been - she spoke beautifully in answer to my questions, said how much she was looking forward to going home for the week-end next day, and clearly had experienced none of the personality changes which Mr Sutcliffe had warned us were a common result of brain injury and surgery. What was stopping Vicky from going home for good was not her brain injury but her poor leg, which had been terribly smashed and still had great metal clamps sticking out of it so that when she practised walking between the parallel bars she had each time to step over the protruding structure with her good leg.

Suddenly Mary called me over to Clare. 'She's just done the most amazing thing', she said excitedly. Ros had again got Clare sitting shakily on the side of the bed and just about managing to hold herself up without tumbling over, Michelle standing behind with hands ready to catch her if she did. Ros had also been talking away to Clare throughout the examination, and when she had got her sitting again she had happened to ask her if she spelt her name with an 'i' or not. Clare had looked at her intently, then without a sound started tracing her name on her knee with the index-finger of her right hand. Needless to say she would not do it again for me, but Ros and Michelle had both seen it and said at once that it was an excellent sign of co-ordination returning.

'Now, Clare, let's get your Daddy doing something useful', said Ros, and while Michelle sat by Clare to support her she went to the cupboard and came back with a balloon, which she got me to blow up not too tightly. Then she said, 'Right now, Clare, Daddy's going to hit this balloon to you and you must hit it back to him. Hit it as hard as you can, Clare!'

I tapped the balloon gently towards her left hand, which was still much the stronger and more active, and with an enormous effort of will she managed to tap it back. We did it several times, and she rarely failed at least to touch the balloon with her hand even if she could not knock it back to me. With the right however she could do little but wave it feebly, so we gave her the satisfaction of a few more goes with the left.

'That's marvellous!' exclaimed Ros, as indeed it was in the context of the last few days, but Clare was now so tired that she was swaying drunkenly and finding it hard to stay sitting up or to keep her head up. But Ros had not finished with her yet. She and Michelle now had Clare standing again, and momentarily at least taking most of her weight with minimal support. 'She's coming along splendidly', said Ros, then suddenly, as they were supporting Clare under each arm to shuffle her to the wheel-chair, she called for help. 'Quick, Peter,' she cried, 'bring the chair round behind her quickly. Clare's collapsing!' Though only fourteen, Clare was a shade taller than Ros and as tall as Michelle, and her sudden dead weight had taken them by surprise. Strong as they were, they were glad when I rapidly pushed the chair up behind Clare and they could lower her into it, now totally exhausted. But what a triumph! Not only had Ros detected the return of the main physical reflexes, however feeble, but we had had our first clear proof that her comprehension and ability to write were intact. The tracing of her name with her finger was quite wonderful. I think that having seen another teenage girl there too had also stimulated Clare to make an effort, for she had watched intently as Vicky had been practising her walking between the parallel bars.

Clare now went to Grosvenor Ward in Garden House, which was an almost new building, having been opened by the Queen, the hospital's patron, less than two years ago. It was a handsome building both inside and out, with its classical facade and beautifully furnished interior, but its air conditioning system was abysmal. This is not unusual. Air conditioning systems are often installed without regard to the partitioning with which the open spaces will subsequently be divided. The result was that on a day like this Grosvenor Ward felt like the tropical house at Kew, and the one poor little desk-top fan perched in one corner was itself almost red-hot with exertion. It made Clare's gas-balloons dance nicely though, and this greatly cheered the two other patients, one a little girl who was leaving that night, the other a tiny baby boy called Jack. Poor little Jack had a bronchial virus of some kind and was coughing rhythmically in a little oxygen tent while his anxious young mother sat with him. The whole of his tiny body would jerk painfully with every cough, but his mother told us he was getting better though he had very nearly died.

The ward-nurse was a very gentle person called Mary, who was everyone's picture of a paediatric nurse. My Mary helped her undress Clare, lift her from the wheel-chair to a sitting position on the bed, then swing her round and lay her down. Nurse Mary then slotted in the 'cot-sides' to the bed so that Clare could not roll out, though the child looked so limp and exhausted from the physiotherapy that I doubted she would stir for hours. Then my Mary went to get some of Clare's things which we had left in our old room opposite the Trauma Unit and I stayed to give the necessary registration details to the nurse, who was starting a new chart and record sheet. Then suddenly, as she looked up from her writing, the nurse cried, 'Look out!', and as I turned to Clare I found she had pulled herself up to a sitting position with both hands on the cot-sides and one leg already half over the top, ready for off!

Clare was now seriously awake, and though still silent and expressionless she drank a chocolate drink through a straw without drawing breath, then demolished a little pot of custard. After that she subsided for a while, but when Frances came in the evening she could hardly believe the difference that twenty-four hours had made. We had quite a stack of new cards for Clare, who watched intently as Frances took each envelope, extracted the card, showed it to her and read out who it was from. Clare then herself picked up an envelope with her left hand, extracted the card with her right hand, scrutinised it intently, and reinserted it in the envelope with complete accuracy. We looked at each other in disbelief. That same right hand, which only four hours ago had not been able to hit a balloon, was now working perfectly.

Parents must try to imagine for themselves what we felt at that moment, and this was not the only surprise Clare had in store for us. Building on the success of my chocolate mousse and little tubs of custard Mary had bought some things called 'Fruit Corners', a great favourite of Clare's. These are small, shallow cartons of yoghurt with a corner separated off for black cherry or strawberry jam or some other flavoursome gunge to mix with it. As Clare seemed to be eyeing these on her bedside table, I took one, peeled the top off, gave it to her in her left hand and put a plastic teaspoon in her right. At first she could not manage it, but after a couple of failures she got one spoonful into her mouth, then another, and a third, but with the fourth she paused, and instead of conveying it to her own mouth she held it out and fed Frances! Mary and I didn't know whether to laugh or cry. It was so magical that we hardly dared speak for fear of breaking the spell.

The strange, solemn face was intent on Frances, but though Frances kept asking her questions - 'Wasn't that delicious?', 'Shall we have another one?' - she could evoke no verbal response until they had polished off a second Fruit Corner together and resumed looking at the cards. At last there was just one left unopened. It was a huge, thick envelope, and having loosened the flap Frances handed it to Clare to open. As before, Clare extracted the contents effortlessly and revealed the most exquisite picture of a bedroom made almost entirely out of pieces of material stuck on a card. There was a little bed with a gorgeous counterpane and a teddy bear propped up against the embroidered pillow, and through the window, which had real curtains, was a beautifully painted view over the fields. It was a real labour of love done by Joanna, another of Clare's artistic friends who used to live next door to us and often 'baby sat' for us. Joanna is a lovely, bubbly young woman of twenty-four, highly artistic but giving up a promising career as a commercial artist to train as a nursery nurse. She must have spent an immense amount of time making this lovely card, and it was certainly appreciated. There was only one teenage expression adequate, and Clare suddenly said it: 'Oh wow!'

CHAPTER NINE

It was about 2 o'clock in the morning when we left Clare sound asleep and went to bed ourselves in a little guest room on the first floor of Garden House. It was one of a very nice suite of three or four bedrooms for parents, with two shower rooms and a large kitchenette-cum-sitting room which was available to all visitors and separated by a locking door from the sleeping quarters. It was a bit of a squeeze in our room, which had only a single bed - and a narrow one at that - but we managed not to fall out and slept fitfully until about 6.30, when we got up and went down to see Clare.

Our minds had been too busy to let us sleep properly, and I was worried that Clare would pull herself up and fall out of bed despite the 'cot-sides'. But finding her still deeply and peacefully asleep we went for a walk in the lovely early morning air and had breakfast in the canteen as soon as it opened. We were its first customers.

By about 7.45 Clare was awake and very thirsty, not surprisingly after a night in a hot-house, for although the temperature in the ward was not as tropical as it had been when we had left her, it was still far too high. We gave her two glasses of orange squash, which she drank eagerly through a straw but still without speaking or even smiling. Then Mary went to buy a few more mousses and boxed drinks for her from the W.H. Smith shop and so missed one of the happiest moments of my life. She had no sooner left the room than a nurse came round with a tea-trolley, popped her head round the door and asked, 'Would you like a cup of tea, Clare?' Not waiting for an answer, which she did not expect, she was just starting to pour her a cup when suddenly, unbelievably, Clare said, 'No, I'm fine, thanks'. It was said perfectly naturally, very politely and with absolute clarity in her usual voice. There was no hesitation or slurring of words whatever. I felt (if Clare will pardon the unflattering analogy) as Balaam must have done when his donkey spoke. I could hardly believe my ears. My only disappointment was that I could not get her to speak again when Mary returned a few minutes later, but Mary could see from my face that something wonderful had happened. I was bursting to tell the Trauma Unit staff too. I knew how anxious they had been about possible damage to the area of the brain responsible for speech, so as soon as Mary was back I dashed across to tell them, pausing only to pick up

W.H. Smith's biggest box of chocolates on the way. I found them in the middle of the change-over from the night to the day staff, and the two night staff, James and Pat, said they would come across and see Clare before they went home. They were as excited as I was, and when they did come over, about half past eight, we all hugged each other with tears in our eyes. Needless to say, Clare would not talk for them but she listened with perplexed intensity, clearly trying to sort out in her mind what on earth had happened and where she was and why. She was also looking very much better, her face less strangely elongated, her neck and jaw less swollen, her eyes looking less as though she had gone ten rounds with a heavyweight boxer, and all the tubes now out except for the catheter, which it was becoming almost impossible to stop her fiddling with. Then about 10 o'clock a member of the neurosurgical team whom we had not seen much of before, a genial, heavily bearded Australian, came to see her and said that this could now come out too. It was like casting off the last hawser from a repaired battleship going out gingerly for trials under its own steam again.

I now had to go home to see to some essential business matters, make some joyful telephone calls to our friends, and deal with the mail, the reams of faxes and the constipated answering machine. But how trivial now seemed some of the matters which had loomed so large only a week ago. It was as though I was seeing life in true perspective for the first time. What price could be put on hearing Clare's 'No, I'm fine, thanks'? What a joy it was to tell Hughie Webb and all our other dear friends! My heart was bursting with joy, and as I knelt again by Clare's bed I found myself praying without words - just focusing my mind on Clare and images of her over the last week, feeling great thankfulness and hope. Then I prayed for Len Davies, for baby Jack in the bed opposite Clare, for all the other patients we had seen and for the staff who looked after them with such skill and devotion. As I said before, I have often found private prayer difficult, but not that day - it just flowed from my mind like a stream into a pool whose depths are unfathomable but whose surface sparkled in the sun, calm, welcoming and wonderfully refreshing.

By the time I returned to the hospital in the early afternoon Clare had had the catheter out and had since performed perfectly. She had tried to get herself out of bed, Mary told me, in sheer determination to go to the toilet properly, and later she had also moved her bowels satisfactorily, for the first time in a week. All systems were 'at go' as the Americans say, and went. She had not, however, spoken again since her polite refusal of a cup of tea early that morning.

As it was another perfect Spring afternoon, sunny and warm and scented with blossom, we took Clare out again to sit in the quiet little garden where she had been with Alice and Charlie the previous day. She watched the helicopter taking off and landing and listened carefully to all our chatter about what it did, but still she said nothing until I told her about speaking to our friend Jenni Dougan, who runs a lovely retirement home at a place called Newlands in the New Forest. Jenni is another of those ageless people who seem to have unlimited energy and are always great fun to be with. Clare thinks the world of her and they chat away to each other like a couple of school friends, though Jenni is old enough to be her mother. I now told Clare that Jenni had invited us all to go and stay with her and she had promised to arrange an all-day ride for her through the forest. I pictured how she could go off in the morning with a girl the same age from a local farm, we could meet them in the car at some prearranged spot for a picnic lunch, then after picnicking and resting the horses they could ride back through the woods. 'So what do you think about that?' I concluded. 'Would you like that?' Clare had no doubts. 'That would be lovely', she replied, and this time Mary heard her. We were so happy.

When we took Clare back to the ward she seemed very tired, but we had no sooner got her out of the wheel-chair and lifted her into bed than she suddenly sat bolt upright, got her legs over the side and was standing up almost before I could reach her. With amazing strength she tried to push me aside and grasped the handle of the broom-cupboard door by the foot of her bed, evidently thinking it was a lavatory-door. She was certainly desperate because it was difficult to unclench her hand from the door-handle and get her into her chair for a trip to the real loo, but we made it without accident and she performed again copiously both ways.

All this may not be the stuff of elevated literature but to find that all the basic bodily functions are working properly was just as important as hearing her speak. The speed of her recovery was now astonishing, though we hardly dared hope that it would become complete. She could eat, drink, walk and talk, and she was continent. But would she be intellectually impaired, would there be psychological problems, would she be able to read and write and go to a normal school again? And would she remain free of infection, or could she still suffer the same sort of relapse as poor Len Davies, who was just about holding his own but still very critically ill?

The grandmother of baby Jack in the oxygen tent opposite was not very consoling when she said that we should all probably catch his bronchial virus as she and Jack's mother and almost all the nurses had it. Certainly they were all choked with coughs and sneezes, and though I could not believe that Clare would have been endangered in that way after all she had been through, I nevertheless mentioned to Sister what the old lady had said. Of course it was nonsense. 'Don't worry', she said. 'Jack's virus is a thing that only attacks babies. It's not communicable to Clare or any of us. What we've all got is just a rotten cold, and I blame this crazy air-conditioning. You'll probably have it tomorrow too,' she added cheerfully, 'though I don't expect Clare will. She's probably built up plenty of resistance while she's been in here'.

After all her exertions Clare ate a splendid supper of baked beans on toast, ice-cream and one of her delicious chocolate mousses, then slept like a log until Frances came about eight o'clock. Frances was thrilled to hear that Clare had spoken so clearly, and though she could not get her to talk again, she witnessed a display of dexterity that was lovely to see. Showing Clare the various gifts that she had been given, I handed her the tin of chocolates which her friend Alice had brought the previous day. They were small, elongated chocolate Easter eggs in twists of purple paper. 'Are you going to keep them for Easter', I asked, 'or hand them round?' Clare considered this carefully for a moment, then holding the tin in her left hand she handed a chocolate egg to each of us in turn and finally took one for herself. This she unwrapped without difficulty, then we all popped our eggs into our mouths together. It was exactly one week from the accident, and not quite six full days from the operation which had removed a piece of her brain.

When we left Clare that night she was for the first time in her old, natural sleeping position, curled up on her side with her faithful Leo the lion and Goodenuff the bear in the crook of her arm. I, however, could not sleep as I had caught the ward's general cold, exactly as Sister had predicted, and in any case my mind was far too busy to rest. So I got up at 6 o'clock, dressed quietly and left Mary fast asleep. Poor Mary. She was exhausted by the strain of the last week, and I was glad to see her having a really good sleep at last.

I tip-toed quietly into the ward to see Clare, who was also fast asleep, and I was delighted to see that baby Jack in his tiny oxygen tent was also much better. His poor little body had been racked with rhythmic coughing for the last two days, but now he was breathing much more easily, coughing only occasionally and a much healthier colour. The night nurse, Justine, kindly made me a cup of tea and we had a pleasant chat. She was a charming person, very petite and so gentle with her often tiny patients like little Jack. Then I decided to drive home for a short time.

It was important to go early because although it was Sunday it was also the day of the London Marathon, which starts on the heath that gives its name to Blackheath where we live. Today it looked like a film set for Tamburlaine, with great pavilions, pleasure domes and portaloos awaiting the cast of thousands of people who would raise thousands of pounds for charity by their sponsored runs. I had to be away again before all the roads round our home were cordoned off about 9 o'clock, but that gave me plenty of time to shower and change, feed the famished fish, send off a few faxes, listen to the answering machine and collect some fresh clothes, including some for Clare too. It was a happier time than my first visit home after the accident. I felt reborn, and the whole house and garden seemed to be rejoicing with me. The garden was thick with narcissi and hyacinths, and even with my cold I was overwhelmed by their beautiful perfume in the sparkling air of that glorious April morning. I thought it must have been the memory of just such a morning as this which inspired Browning's 'Oh, to be in England'.

I was back well before nine to find Clare's bed curtained off with Mary helping to wash her within.

'Hi, Clare', I called, 'it's Daddy. But I'm not allowed to come in'.

'Hi, Dad!', came the reply, then Mary's face looked out with the happiest of smiles. 'Isn't it wonderful?', she said.

It was indeed, but feeling a huge sneeze coming on I fled the room and went to regale myself on an extra large breakfast of bacon and eggs in the canteen. I felt so happy I even felt like hugging the extraordinarily sour-faced cashier at the till but settled for an ineffective smile and a polite 'Good Morning' instead. In treating myself to such a heroic breakfast I was acting on the principle 'Feed a cold and starve a fever', but as I reached the toast and marmalade stage it suddenly occurred to me that that prescription had a Delphic ambiguity. At face value the injunction seems to be that you should feed yourself if you have a cold but starve yourself if you have a fever; but giving a slightly different cadence to the sentence could equally well imply that if you feed a cold you will thereafter have a fever, which you will then have to starve! Language is a complex business, and for brains subtle enough to handle it to be strong enough to survive the battering that Clare's had had seems truly miraculous. Yet we are asked to believe that they just 'evolved' accidentally without a divine plan. Who could possibly look into the heavens or down a microscope and not believe in a divine intelligence? It is beyond all reason, and reason, God knows, is all we have to go on.

Clare was now moved out of the four-bedded ward into a little single room of her own. Besides having the luxury of its own toilet and shower *en suite,* which would be much more convenient for her, it was a lovely, light room with its previous occupant's jolly paper flowers still on the wall. It was also next to a big general ward and community room accommodating about ten or twelve children's beds around three outside walls, the inside wall being glass and running the full length of the corridor. There was a staff desk by this inner wall and a huge play and television area in the middle. It would be nice for Clare to be wheeled in to join them when she was stronger and able to be more sociable. Some of the children there were mobile, but the majority were not. Vicky, who had had the same operation as Clare a few weeks earlier, was normally in there but had gone home for the week-end. Most of the other children were much younger, but there was one other teenager, a very cheerful young lady of about Clare and Vicky's age called Hester. Though she was flat on her back in a plaster cast after an operation to correct some malformation of her spine, her bed was on wheels and the nurses moved her around so that she could watch a video or play cards with Vicky. She was the life and soul of the ward, full of fun and teenage prattle. Happily her operation had gone well and she could look forward to a full recovery.

Among the younger children was a little boy of seven who had had the same operation as Vicky and Clare, but poor Terry was still not able to swallow seven months after his accident, and when we saw him sitting in his wheelchair still being fed through a nose-tube we realised how very lucky both Clare and Vicky had been. Yet he was a brave little chap, and I later discovered from the physios that they had good hopes of getting him to swallow before much longer. Apparently he was swallowing in his sleep but not when he was awake. His parents told me he had been playing 'chicken' with some other lads - running across the road in front of cars.

The tiny tots were in separate wards on the other side of Garden House, and among the sad sights there were some cheerful little characters. One exquisitely pretty little girl of about four was in plaster from her waist down, having had a third and final operation to correct a malformed pelvis. She had beautiful golden curls, and as she looked as though she might fly out of the window at any moment to look for Peter Pan, the staff called her Tinkerbell. Then there was little Amy, a child who had spent most of her young life either there or in Great Ormond Street Children's Hospital. I never found out what was wrong with her, but she kept having to go for operations in Great Ormond Street and back to the London for convalescence. Every time she went home something went wrong, and I think she now regarded Garden House as her home. She certainly had a proprietorial air as she played nurses up and down the corridors, and was a real 'character', much loved by the staff. God only knows what the future will hold for her and some of those other children. It was pitiful to see how some of them were suffering, but pity alone is useless. What they need and get from the staff is encouragement and cheerfulness, and they respond with a courage that is often quite astounding.

Clare was very tired after her move to her new room, and after every little exertion she would fall into a deep sleep; but it was now a healing, healthy, natural sleep, not the motionless coma of her time in the Trauma Unit. She was unfortunately fast asleep and unstirrable when Moira and Angela popped over from Trauma to see her, but she woke up when the Bulmer family arrived in the late morning - Philip, Denyse, the fourteen-year-old Caroline and five-year-old Jack. Phil and Denyse knew better than anyone what we had been going through after their own experiences with their spastic daughter Louise, and there was an unspoken understanding between us when I shook my old friend's hand. In the meantime the irrepressible Carrie was chattering away non-stop to Clare, who would normally have been chattering back simultaneously as teenage girls do, but she was silent now, though listening intently. Carrie had brought Clare a gorgeous teddy bear holding the string of a gas-filled balloon with a smiling yellow sun on it. Clare loved it and clearly loved Carrie's chatter too, but try as she would she was so sleepy that she could not keep her eyes open for long. She soon showed, however, that she was not switched off. As Carrie babbled on about her favourite subject, clothes - she was dressed in psychedelic spangled tights and a bizarre T-shirt - and wondered aloud which market was better, Kennington or Camden, Clare opened one eye and said sleepily but decisively, 'Camden for clothes'. Phil looked away and wiped his eyes. It was bringing back painful memories for him, his joy at Clare's recovery being tinged with sadness that his hopes for Louise had not been fulfilled. Mary and I felt for Phil and Denyse, just as they felt for us. No-one can possibly know what our sort of experiences are like until he has gone through it.

In the afternoon Joanna came in and Clare was thrilled to see her. Her beautiful hand-made card had pride of place on the window sill, but she had brought another, even lovelier one. Clare was entranced and gazed at it for a good two minutes before announcing in her strange, solemn way, 'It's lovely'. Clare made a brave fight against her sleepiness while Jo was there, but fell fast asleep again the moment she had gone. She was clearly exhausted by all the excitement because she would still not give her beloved Frances the joy of hearing her speak when she popped in an hour later. But I was in for a real surprise in the early evening after Frances had left. Mary had gone out of the room to make some phone calls and I was alone with an apparently comatose Clare when she suddenly sat up and said, 'I want the toilet, *quickly* !'

She was already trying to lower the cot-rail so that she could get out of bed, and as there was no nurse about I got her to swing her legs out and put her arms round my neck, then I lifted her up until she was standing and we shuffled backwards together into the toilet and sat her down. Putting her hands on the side-rails I told her to be sure to hold on tight, then rushed off down the corridor to the front desk, where I found Sister and brought her back with me. Then as I waited outside the toilet I rejoiced to hear an indignant Clare saying politely but firmly, 'I can wipe myself, thank you'. I could not help laughing, but a few moments later she had an even better surprise in store for me. For out she came under her own steam - walking unsupported for the first time, with Sister just behind ready to catch her if she faltered. She made it to the bed and collapsed into it. She could walk!

That night we rang our friends and relatives excitedly with this marvellous news, then ourselves had an early night for once. Clare was clearly exhausted by her exertions, and I was feeling rotten with my cold. But we were worried that Clare might try to get out of bed herself in the night and fall, so we asked Sister if Mary could perhaps have a mattress so that she could sleep on the floor next to Clare's bed (the other side being against the wall). Sister was delighted at the suggestion and provided not just a mattress but a proper folding camp-bed and beautifully crisp, white sheets and pillow-cases. It gave us all peace of mind.

After leaving Clare and Mary to settle down for the night in her room I went across to the deserted Chapel before turning in myself in the guest-room upstairs. As I sat there with just the little altar light burning I thought over all that had happened in the last week. There was so much to be thankful for. This time only a week ago Clare was being kept alive by machines, her brain dangerously swollen, and we had been told that she would have to undergo surgery. Today she had walked by herself. Tonight I could sleep soundly. But others would be waiting anxiously for news in the ITU Relatives' Room or on the two stacking chairs outside the theatre corridor, and poor Len Davies was barely alive. My prayers went out to them all, and I felt very privileged to be in a great hospital like this where God-given skills were being so ably dedicated to the work of healing.

CHAPTER TEN

Monday morning started with an accident as poor Clare evacuated in bed about 7 o'clock even though Mary said she had been to the toilet only two hours before. She seemed distressed and rather groggy, but she perked up when Mary and I stripped the bed and her and gave her a nice shower. She was still too groggy to worry about her natural modesty: she let me hold her up while Mary showered her, then we put her in a clean, dry pair of pyjamas and sat her in the wheelchair while we changed the bed. The nurses had brought us fresh sheets but we told them not to worry about making the bed. It was nice for us to have something useful to do, and they were very busy with the rising and shining of many little ones.

As soon as the bed was re-made, Clare immediately tried to get into it and kept saying, 'I'm so tired, I'm so tired'. We therefore helped her back to bed, but before letting her lie down Mary insisted on combing her hair. Then the most extraordinary thing happened. Mary was gathering her hair to put it in a pony-tail with a little elastic toggle when Clare raised both hands, pushed her gently away, then taking the hair in her left hand put the toggle on effortlessly with her right. There was no fumbling or second attempt. The whole complex action - which I tried myself and could not do - was performed perfectly first time, the fingers of her right hand deftly doubling the toggle back on itself to halve its size and hold the pony-tail tight. I could hardly believe my eyes.

Fearing that Clare might get out of bed and fall if no-one was with her, Mary and I determined that one or other of us would be with her all the time from now on, day and night. We would take it in turns to go for meals, and at night Mary would continue to sleep on the camp-bed beside Clare. As she was still sleeping a lot of the time we were able to read business papers, write letters and notes and generally keep our work ticking over, but I also amused myself - and them too, I hope - by writing a daily bulletin, as from Clare, to the staff of the Trauma Unit. I took these bulletins over early each morning and left them together with a box of chocolates or biscuits on the table just outside the Unit. I wrote the first that Monday morning while Clare was so very sleepy:

Hi everyone, it's Clare. I thought I'd drop you a line to let you know how I'm getting on. I know I'm in hospital now and Dad and Mum told me I had an accident and an operation on my head, but I can't remember anything about it. Worse still, they keep talking about all of you, saying how marvellous you all are and how well you looked after me, but I can't remember being in the Trauma Unit at all! Dad says it only means I have the unusual pleasure of meeting for the first time the best friends I ever had. It does feel odd though!

Actually, I'm a bit worried about Dad and Mum. Every time I say something they look as though they're going to burst into tears, and they won't leave me alone for a minute. I can't even go to the loo without them. It's a bit much! Dad also has a bad cold, refuses to kiss me 'goodnight' and rushes out of the room every few minutes to sneeze. He collided with the tea trolley yesterday and nearly broke all the cups! In between sneezes he keeps giving me presents and promising me treats. He even bought me a new camera the other day for when I eventually go on my exchange visit to Italy - I'd have been there now but for my accident. I'm going to send him over for a brain scan if he goes on like this. Still, make hay while the sun shines, say I, and if he wants to get writer's cramp in his cheque-writing hand, who am I to stop him ?

One thing that Dad and Mum keep saying and which makes me think they're not so crazy after all is that you lot are the most fantastic group of young people they've ever been privileged to meet. The trouble is, I haven't met you all yet. I'll get over one day and say 'hello' as soon as I can, and if any of you are passing Garden House on your way home, do pop in. It was great to meet James and Pat, but I'm sorry I was asleep when Angela and Moira popped in. I asked

Dad what they were like and he said, 'Perfect combinations of brains and beauty'. I think Dad's getting a bit susceptible in his middle age!

See you soon and lots of love to you all,
Clare.

About mid-morning Clare had the stitches out of her long operation wound that ran right across her forehead, but they decided to leave the stitches for a bit longer in the place where the drain had been at the back, which was still a bit 'squelchy'. Then the Chaplain popped in to see us with a lovely book for her called *The Velveteen Rabbit*. Sadly it is out of print, for it is a truly delightful and unobtrusively allegorical story about a much loved fluffy toy rabbit who eventually became real. It is very much in the tradition of C.S. Lewis, whose Narnia stories Clare can almost recite verbatim. She listened avidly to this new story and kept asking for it to be repeated. It was almost as though she was five or six again. Every time I thought she had gone off to sleep and stopped reading, a reproachful eye would open and demand resumption. Sometimes too she would listen for hours to the taped stories which we had brought in for her to the Trauma Unit, *Kim, Black Beauty* and the Narnia stories being her favourites.

After a light lunch reinforced by some ice-cream which Mary had brought we dressed Clare for her physiotherapy session and wheeled her over to the gym. As before, the staff had carefully arranged that Vicky would be there at the same time, and there is no doubt that this was good stimulation for Clare as well as teenage companionship for them both. Nigel was there too, already doing his vigorous exercises and full of fun as usual. There was an advertisement for trainee physiotherapists on the notice-board, and I asked Nigel jokingly if he was going to apply as he would be superbly well qualified by experience on the receiving end.

'I tried', he replied in the middle of about a hundred press-ups, 'but they said I was far too experienced to be a trainee. They want someone totally inexperienced, and in fact they've had an applicant from among the newly unemployed.'

'Who's that?', I asked.

'Neil Kinnock', came the reply. I should have guessed! It was just after the General Election when the Labour Party had lost.

While I was chatting to Nigel, Vicky had taken out a pack of cards and was setting out an immensely complicated-looking 'patience': no intellectual impairment there evidently! Clare in the meantime was having her reflexes tested on a bed, then she was helped to sit up. The difference from last Friday was astonishing. Then she had not been able to lift her head up without help, and she could only feebly hit a balloon with one hand. Now she could sit bolt upright and play the balloon game with each hand alternately, 'five to Daddy, five to Mummy', and so on. Next she was made to sit on a big ball, with support, to try to regain balance, and she was able to climb the steps to the dais one at a time (with the added stimulation of seeing Vicky doing her walking between the parallel bars). Ros and her team were as delighted with her progress as we were, but it was a very exhausted Clare whom we wheeled back to Garden House an hour later.

She went to sleep on her visitors in the afternoon, but in the evening, after supper, she suddenly came to life with a vengeance. It must have been about 9 o'clock that she woke up from a heavy doze and pulled herself upright in bed. Thinking that she wanted the toilet we let the side rail down, she swung her legs out and we helped her to stand. But instead of going into the toilet, she pushed me aside and marched out into the corridor. Mary and I followed supporting her, afraid she would fall but fascinated to see what she would, and could, do.

When we asked her what she wanted and where she was going she would not reply, nor had she spoken at all since she woke up, but it soon became clear that she wanted a good look round. I suppose she was still trying to come to terms with where she was. We helped her to walk round the corridor, peering into the now darkened wards, until she came to Sister's desk, where Dr Britto happened to be sitting writing a few notes after seeing another neurosurgical patient. He was as fascinated as we were, and when Clare got hold of the telephone and we tried to make her put it down, he signed to us to leave her alone.

With amazing precision Clare began pressing numbers and Mary spotted that she was trying to ring her friend Joanna, who had made her the two beautiful cards. Mary recognised the number, but Clare could not get the number and the code in the right sequence and after several goes lost concentration and began pressing all the buttons indiscriminately in an outburst of frustration. At that we did stop her,

but Dr Britto was bubbling over with delight. 'Marvellous!' he said.
'Just the right reaction for a teenager, to get on the telephone as soon
as possible! Believe me, seeing this sort of thing makes it all
worthwhile - all the twenty-four hour shifts and weekends on call.
Good girl, Clare! You'll be ringing your friends and boosting your
Dad's phone bill soon enough!'

It was still some time before we could get the hyperactive Clare
settled, but eventually she fell into an exhausted sleep and I amused
myself writing 'her own' account of the day's exploits to the Trauma
Unit, to be delivered the next morning with a celebratory, poly-
saturated chocolate cake bulging with arteriosclerotic double cream.

> Hi again, it's Clare. I'm feeling so much better. I
> sat up for breakfast yesterday and had a really good
> shower. Dad and Mum still behave very oddly.
> They seemed to think there was something clever
> about my making a pony-tail, holding my hair in my
> left hand and slipping a little coloured toggle on with
> my right. I think they're getting a bit senile! Then
> Dad went potty when he left the room for a minute
> (he simply won't leave me alone) and I got out of bed
> and went to the loo. What does he expect me to do -
> wet the bed?!

> In the afternoon I met a new pal called Vicky, who's
> my age, when we went to the gym. Vicky
> slaughtered the phyios at cards, while I was made to
> do very odd things - walking up and down a flight of
> steps that led nowhere, sitting on a big coloured ball
> (made me feel a bit wobbly), walking up and down
> the room, then knocking a balloon to Dad and Mum,
> five times to each with each hand. Boy, did I make
> them run! Mum's good at ball games but too fat.
> Dad's just useless. It was a hoot!

> I must say I felt very tired afterwards, and oddly
> enough I couldn't quite get my name and address
> right when they asked me to write it down. Still, I
> nearly did. I slept the Sleep of the Just (a corny joke

of Dad's - he then says, 'the Just Exhausted'), then
some friends rocked up - my pal Frances (Dad and
Mum's goddaughter, who's a silversmith) and
Doreen, who's sixty-seven but seems like seventeen
and drives a sports car. I was so sleepy, I couldn't
chat much, and I'm afraid that after a bit I had to
say, 'I'm sorry, I'm going to have to go to sleep',
and I did. They'd gone when I woke up, so I got out
of bed. Dad and Mum tried to stop me, but I took no
notice and walked down the corridor to the front
desk, where I saw a Dr Britto who seemed pleased to
see me. He seemed to know me, but I couldn't
remember him. Anyway, I tried to use the phone to
ring my friends, but I somehow couldn't get Jo's
number right and couldn't get through. Dad didn't
help. (He's rotten about the phone - always moaning
about the bills, yet he gasses on for hours about
boring business to his own friends). I then walked
round the wards, saw the other children, got some
very funny looks from people and went back to my
own room, with Mum and Dad still in tow. (I simply
can't get rid of them). Oh, I forgot to say I had my
stitches out at the front though not at the back, where
I've got a bit of a squelchy lump which they fussed
about for a bit. Anyway, I haven't got a temperature
so they didn't seem too worried.

Sorry I'm having to get Dad to act as scribe yet
again. You'll all qualify for top jobs in MI6's
cryptographic service if you can decipher his scribble
- or you could take it down to the Pharmacy and see
what they make up from it! Mum's insisted on
sleeping on a camp bed next to mine in case I try and
get out in the night and fall - just as if! Dad still has
his cold, won't give me a kiss and keeps rushing out
of the room every time he feels a sneeze coming on.
I really think they'd be better off in a home
sometimes... Anyway, Dad seems to know what the
Charts are at last. He's such a Square (or would be

112

if he wasn't so round!) that he used to think charts
were only what admirals have in their cabins on
ships. But he's improving (amazingly). I was talking
about what was in the Charts to my friend Joanna
when he suddenly piped up and said that the Trauma
Group were at the top of his Charts, no. 1, for the
rest of his life, and Mum agreed.

I'll be along to see you all soon I hope. Angela
popped in yesterday and I was asleep again! But
Dad, intelligent for once, woke me up so I could say
'hello'. Looking forward to seeing the rest of you
too. Dad and Mum keep hugging each other - they're
a bit embarrassing really, at their age. Dad said the
best hug he ever had was in the Trauma Unit from
one of you called Sandra, and Mum - instead of
fetching him one round the ear with her handbag -
agreed! I think I've been missing something, but I
can't properly get the hang of what it is. Well, must
go for now. Lots of love,

Clare.

X X X X X ⟵—————— Power hugs!

V.I.P.S.
Dad says that one day last week you had a staff photo
taken in the Unit because Jan was leaving. Could I
please have a copy? An enlargement, if poss. I've
got Dad to cough up a fiver (enclosed) but if it's not
enough we'll get him to cough up some more (and if
he has any problem coughing up I'll send for Linda
and get her to give him one of her wiggly-worm
specials!)

Happily the 'wiggly worms' were creatures of the past. Now that
she was much more active Clare could cough up the much reduced
amounts of phlegm and fluid from her lungs without the aid of suction
tubes, and luckily she did not catch the streaming cold that I and

almost all the staff had. She was improving rapidly every day now on the physical side, and when we went to the gym the next day, which was Tuesday, Ros told us that we must begin to exercise her mind and get her writing. 'You must push her hard', said Ros, 'just as we do here in the gym. Her mind needs as much physio as her body now'. So in the days that followed we made little tests and quizzes for Clare and it was wonderful to see her mind recovering just as her body was doing.

'Recovery', however, is relative. To us, who had seen Clare at her worst, her progress was astounding. To see her eating and drinking by herself, beginning to be able to walk short distances unaided, talking fairly coherently and doing such intricate things as putting a toggle on a pony-tail was so wonderful for us that we tended to forget how terrible she must still appear to anyone who had not seen her since before the accident. Mary's mother, though very brave about it, was clearly distressed when she came to see Clare today for the first time, and I could only be thankful that we had dissuaded her from coming before. But I am blest with a super mother-in-law, despite the inevitable jokes that I put into 'Clare's' bulletin of the day's events to amuse the Trauma Unit the following morning:

> Buongiorno! It's me again, Clare, who should have been in Italy with my school friends on an exchange. When I was in the gym yesterday Ros asked me if I learnt any foreign languages. I couldn't remember at first, but when she asked if I did French, I knew at once I didn't and said 'No!' I *hated* French and gave it up. The trouble is I was so tired after playing ping-pong and walking up and down the stairs that lead nowhere (one has to humour the physios but I don't see the point of it myself) that I couldn't remember that I did Italian. Anyway, when Dad reminded me, I said 'Buongiorno', which they seemed to think was very clever (but then again they're all a bit thick, so you have to make allowances!). But seriously, you really should shine a light in Dad's eyes or feel his bumps. He's still behaving very oddly. I say the simplest things and he seems so pleased, not his usual grumpy self at all.

For instance, yesterday I didn't want all my cup of
tea because I'd had a big glass of orange, and when
he asked if I minded if he finished it and I said, 'No,
of course not', he did a little dance. (I wondered if
he'd been drinking, but surely not so early in the
morning.)

It was a busy day. My Gran, Mum's mum, came
down from Cambridge with lots of presents but sat in
a bit of a stodge and Dad started getting irritable with
Mum. I think Gran is getting a bit more reconciled
to Dad now he and Mum have been married twenty-
four years, but even so Dad was getting up a head of
steam over something Gran said. Mum once told me
he had set his relationship with Gran back to square
one when they'd been married five years and Gran
suggested she might give them a washing-up machine
for their anniversary present. Dad had said, 'No,
thanks, you gave me a very good one five years ago
and it still functions perfectly!' Male chauvinist!
Anyway it was a long time before I was born.

Two of my school friends popped in. It was nice to
see them - more fun than boring old Dad and Mum!
And Michelle came down from Trauma. It was
lovely to meet another one of you. Dad teased her
about her new glasses and pretended not to recognise
her! Oh, and I nearly forgot to tell you, I had a
lovely, lovely bath in the morning full of bubble-
stuff. It felt so nice. It was the first proper bath I'd
had.

In the afternoon it was gym again, as I said, and I
tried to play ping-pong with Vicky. I managed to hit
the ball, but that was about all. She was very patient
with me, but I'm no good at table tennis anyway.
Still, it was fun. Gran went home after that. It had
been lovely to see her, and we all had great big hugs.
Then when Dad came back from seeing her into a

taxi I'd finished my gym, and because it was starting to rain Dad and Mum decided to wheel me back by the underground passages. Needless to say we got lost in the labyrinth, and I half expected to see the Minotaur any minute. He'd have had no difficulty finding us as Dad and Mum started rowing as they always do in the car, arguing about navigation. They carry on like characters in Russian novels. Parents!! But you know what they're like.

I was so tired when we got back that I just wanted to curl up and go to sleep, but I was glad when Dad bullied me into eating my supper. Frances came too, then as Dad needed to go home to see to messages and feed our fish he took Frances with him. But Mum hadn't told him properly where she had left the car after picking Gran up from the station in the morning. He couldn't find it for ages, and he and Frances got wet through in a thunderstorm. I bet he was apoplectic! Anyway, I'll hear all about it from Frances.

Lots of love,

Clare.

P. S. You should see how glam I am! Dad has a fabulous line in cousins up in Lancashire. I got a gigantic parcel today from his cousin Dorothy, who has a dress-shop. It was full of gorgeous things, including a pale green night-dress made of pure silk and a pair of dainty white slippers with ostrich feathers round the edges. Dad says he'll borrow them to go and rescue Andromeda, but I don't know what he means.

P.P.S. Dad's cold is a bit better now and as he's no longer rushing out every five minutes to sneeze and knock tea-trolleys over I'm worried that he's not getting enough exercise. I'm going to ask Ros for a punishing programme of aerobics for him, and if the cold settles on his chest I'll call in Linda with the wigglies!

CHAPTER ELEVEN

The next day, Wednesday, just nine days after her operation, Clare showed us clearly for the first time that she had not lost the ability to write properly. So far we had had the extraordinary tracing of her signature with her finger on the first day in the gym before she could even talk, but her first attempt to write with a pen on a piece of paper the previous day had been a frustrated series of capital letters scrunched up on the right side of the paper, as though she did not see the left half. She would try to write a word then get stuck and repeat the same letter, usually 'E', again and again. Today, however, I made up a little form for her to fill in saying 'Name, 'Address', 'Telephone number' and 'Signature', and I gave it to her casually as a form the hospital had asked her to complete. Curiously her name was just a jumble of capital letters, as was her signature. It looked in fact as though she had been trying to write the word 'signature'. Her address, however, was absolutely correct, though written in capital letters, and she had got her telephone number right too. Then I took another sheet of paper and suggested we should write a note to her Italian exchange friend who had sent her a lovely card. This time she began correctly in the top left with 'I wish' in small as well as capital letters but in a very big, unformed, childish hand. But then she got stuck, and again a whole series of disjointed capital letters came out and she threw down the pen in frustration.

'Never mind', I said, 'it will soon come back. I'll write the note for you if you like, then you can sign it.'

Taking a fresh sheet of paper I wrote 'I wish I could come and stay with you. I received your lovely card'. Then I gave her the paper and pen and suggested that she should add a note of thanks, then sign it. To my surprise and delight she wrote immediately and correctly 'Thanks a lot', but when I said, 'Now sign it nicely', she had a complete block.

She glared at the paper for about two minutes with fearful concentration, poised her pen several times, but simply could not do it. Mary thought it might help if we showed her our own signatures, so I took a separate sheet and said 'Let's all sign our names on this'. I signed mine first, then Mary signed hers, then Clare signed hers, absolutely naturally and without a moment's hesitation.

It was fascinating, almost eerie, to see Clare's faculties returning - like a flower opening unevenly or a whole series of curtains being drawn back. The order in which the faculties returned was also curious. At a time when she had no difficulty in recognising words or geometrical shapes, she was still having problems with colours, being unable to distinguish blue, brown and black for quite a long time after she could not only identify circles, triangles, squares and so forth but correctly write their names. She also came out with extraordinary Malapropisms. Sometimes she was completely unaware of having said the wrong word, particularly when she was tired, but increasingly she realised her inability always to find the right word and tried to avoid embarrassment either by not initiating conversation or, if she could not answer a question about someone's name or an event, by covering up. She would use a little series of stock phrases, such as 'It's a secret' or 'I shan't tell you' or 'You *know* what she's called'. And sometimes she would just lie down and say, 'I've had enough, I'm going to sleep!'

The next day, Maundy Thursday, I started writing little quizzes for her to complete. First I asked her to fill in the same 'form' as yesterday - name, address, telephone number and signature, but this time I added 'Name of school' just before 'Signature'. She did this correctly and without hesitation. Then I asked her to copy out three sentences which I had written out for her: 'My name is Clare and I am in hospital after an accident. I banged my head and had to have an operation. But I am getting better now'. She did this reasonably well, though she missed out three words and had difficulty in judging how many words she could get on a line, as she scrunched words up at the right-hand edge. But it was legible and was also getting the message through to her about where she was and why, as she was by no means always able to answer that question, or may not have wanted to. Then I wrote a list of six of her good friends' first names and asked her to copy them out. To my astonishment she wrote instead, absolutely correctly, not the first names but the surnames of five out of the six.

The day after that we were more ambitious. I wrote the names of some of C.S. Lewis's Narnia books, which are great favourites, plus the titles of two Shakespeare plays which she knows, and in each case I left a word out for Clare to fill in. But she could do only one of them, 'The Lion, the Witch and the _____ ', and even though she got 'Wardrobe' she confused the letters 'b' and 'd' exactly as she had done when first learning to read and write. The next quiz, however, about colours, she got completely right. It began with 'The traffic lights go Red, then _____, then _____ ', and she correctly filled in 'yellow' and 'green'. She then added the right colours in 'The sea is blue', 'Grass is green' and 'My hair is brown'. Her writing was also firm and clear, so unlike the tortured letters of the words she had struggled to write in the book-names quiz I had given her. Oddly, however, while she had no hesitation in writing the correct colours in these little sentences, she still could not reliably distinguish the colours herself when asked to name the colour of something in the room.

A shapes test presented no problem. She wrote 'square', 'circle' and 'triangle' without hesitation against the corresponding shapes, and spelt them correctly too. She could also fill in the right answers to 2 x 2, 2 x 3, 2 x 4 and 2 x 5, but 5 x 5 came next and she wrote 50 instead of 25. Finally I gave her three sentences to copy out, this time about Good Friday, which it was. 'Today is called Good Friday. It is the day when Jesus was crucified. He rose again from the dead on Easter Sunday. We open Easter eggs then to celebrate his coming to life again'. Though some of the words were difficult, Clare wrote it out with much more confidence and accuracy than the simpler sentences of the previous day. Her handwriting too had more character: though still a big, round hand, the letters were now recognisably in Clare's style, and she had no trouble today with spacing out words on a line. The faculty we take for granted of gauging the distance to the end of a line so that the last word will either fit comfortably or be saved for the next line had now returned.

Another day, and she was better again. Easter Saturday's arithmetic quiz was much more difficult involving all four functions: 2 x 2, 2 + 2, 6 ÷ 3, 3 + 3, 4 + 2, 8 + 4, 10 - 5, 100 - 50, 10 + 2, 2 x 5. But it was only on 8 + 4 that she even paused before writing the correct answers. Then I had written out three questions requiring her to read a short text:

'Jim bought four kilos of peaches and there were four peaches to the kilo. How many peaches did he buy?'

'The peaches were 50 pence each. How much did they cost?'

'Jim gave the shopkeeper £10. How much change did he get?'

It is strange how the questions I expected her to find more difficult proved easy for her, and vice versa. I had expected her to struggle with these three, but on the contrary she wrote in the answers immediately, as though her brain had been working them out automatically as she read the questions. Perhaps it was the practical and visual nature of these questions that made it easier - questions about real things that could be visualised rather than numbers in the abstract.

Finally there was a little quiz about school. I wrote down the names of twelve subjects and asked her to say whether she studied them or not by writing 'yes' or 'no' against each one. This she also did correctly, though when she had been asked to say which subjects she did, she had not been able to do it spontaneously. Interesting too was the fact that her distant memory was better than her recent one. When asked to give her class-teacher's name, she gave the teacher of the previous, not the current, year. Similarly when asked how many pets she had, she wrote '2 x bird, 1 x fish', but she now had only one bird, the other having died over a year ago.

While Mary and I were working on Clare's intellectual rehabilitation, the physios were working wonders for her physically in the gym. She now began her sessions lying on her back, bringing up her knees, then raising and lowering her stomach a dozen times while keeping her shoulders on the ground. Then with knees bent and stomach up she had to stretch out first one leg, then the other, five times each. (I tried it too and found it marvellous for tightening the tummy muscles!). Then lying full length on her side and keeping her legs straight she had to raise the upper leg and swing it backwards and forwards as far as it would go. Then there were the balloon and ball games, the steps and a most formidable exercise for balance and co-ordination where she began by sitting on a big ball then had to 'walk' herself forward till she was lying horizontally on it. This of course needed a lot of support, but she was determined to manage it and had complete trust that Ros would not let her fall.

I cannot speak too highly of the work of the physiotherapists in the neurosurgical gym, and I was horrified to hear recently that it had been closed, leaving the physios to try to do the best they can without space or equipment on the wards. It was a 'cost-cutting' exercise, but how many administrators and cost-cutters have themselves been cut out I wonder. These specialised units and their esprit de corps are not created overnight but can be destroyed in seconds by the stroke of an accountant's pen. Neurosurgical rehabilitation is immensely specialised. We saw the physios in action not just with Clare but with several other patients who happened to be there at the same times. We saw a nameless man they called 'Robert' because he seemed to respond best to it. No-one knew who he was, nor had any relatives or friends reported him missing. He had been walking out of a pub when he was struck on the head by the wing mirror of a passing lorry. He could not speak and was in a terrible state when we first saw him - just as Clare had been when she first went to the gym, head sunk on chest, unable to straighten up let alone stand. He had a nose tube inserted, catheter and quite a lot of 'wiring'. But when we next saw him, only three days later, he was transformed - able to stand with help, holding his head up, shaking it in sheer frustration that he could not yet speak (and Robert was obviously not his name) but clearly well on the way to what promised to be a high degree of recovery. Then there was Rose, a dear old lady whose right side was semi-paralysed. The girls were so nice to the dear old soul as she struggled to throw a beanbag with the weak hand, and when Mary made her a cup of tea while she was waiting for the porters to come after her session, she said with a nod towards Clare and Vicky, 'It doesn't matter so much for me, I've had my life. But thank God they can do something for these young ones, God bless them'.

It was so nice that parents were encouraged to help and be with their children as much as possible. As the Easter week-end was coming up, Ros was keen that we should learn the exercise routine for Clare and keep her at it. We were only too pleased to be involved, and as I practised the exercises with Clare I found muscles I did not know I had. But it almost caused me to end up in the Trauma Unit myself one day. Having been kneeling to support Clare as she did her physical jerks one day in her room, I stood up suddenly and gave my head a terrific crack on the edge of a TV stand which protruded from the wall at a height of less than six feet from the ground. It was the daftest thing. It was at the end of a rigid arm sticking out of the wall just by the door to the lavatory, exactly at the level of Clare's forehead, and I had been constantly afraid that she might bang her head on it as she went to the toilet. Happily it was my head and not hers which got the bang. I really saw stars, and a nurse who was coming in at that very moment said 'Ouch, I heard that! Sit on the bed for a minute and I'll be right back'. When she returned, however, it was not with a bottle of aspirins and a soothing cup of tea

as I had fondly hoped, but a complaints form. 'Just sign this and I'll
fill it in', she said triumphantly. 'We've been trying to get rid of that
stupid thing for ages. This is the only way to get things done!' And
sure enough, that same afternoon two very large men with two
enormous bags of tools came and took the thing down. Anyone would
have thought they were going to dismantle the whole hospital, not do
something that needed five minutes with a screw driver.

As it was Easter week Clare had a whole warren of chocolate
bunnies and a positive hatchery of chocolate eggs. She had cards all
over the walls, and every visitor and every post added to her store.
Then on Good Friday there was a special treat in store. Clare by now
was able to join the other children in the big ward, where she could be
wheeled to sit with Vicky or with Hester, the girl who was lying flat
on her back in a plaster. Sometimes they chatted - especially Hester,
who was the life and soul of the ward - and sometimes they watched a
video on the television. But on Good Friday there was live
entertainment as the Royal Navy paid a visit in the persons of a
contingent from HMS Vincent.

It was a delight to see the children's faces as the ABs and WRENS
marched in, tremendously smart in their immaculate uniforms and
dishing out huge piles of chocolate eggs to all the children. The
Commander and his wife came too, and when she came round to see
Clare she recognised the frontal lobotomy scar and told us that her
daughter had had the same operation. In her case, though, it had not
been as a result of an accident but to cure the most terrible epilepsy.
It had been a last resort but a complete success. Her daughter, now
eighteen, was totally free from fits, mentally unimpaired in any way
and learning to drive a car.

All the children in Garden House who had been able to do so had
gone home for the week-end, and Vicky had gone home for good the
previous day. Her parents had come for her about 10 o'clock, but
before they left there was a treat in store for her too. Vicky and her
younger brother were taken up to the helipad and shown the inside of
the helicopter which had brought her in and saved her life. She was
thrilled, and though it would still be several weeks before the
machinery could be taken out of the badly shattered leg, it was only a
matter of time before she would be able to walk properly again. The
great thing was that she was fully recovered mentally, and a few days
later we were thrilled to see a photograph of her playing her cello in

the *Daily Express,* the newspaper which has so generously sponsored the London Hospital's helicopter. In the meantime, as I shook her father's hand I saw the happiest man in the world. God grant that Clare would do as well. So far she was doing well, but we had seen from Len Davies how quickly something could go wrong and we kept trying to curb our growing optimism.

There was little change in Len's condition but at least he was still alive. Mary and Carole had coffee and a talk together every day, and despite all her own problems Carole kept popping in to say 'hello' to Clare and brought her the most lovely little teddy bear wearing a smart bow tie. The biggest worry about Len was that his kidneys were not working at all, and he was surviving only by dialysis. If they did not start working soon the future would be very bleak even if he did survive. But still I felt in my heart that he would pull through. I had known it when I had sat in the Chapel in one of our darkest hours, and I told Carole so. It was to be another ten days before he began to improve, but he did, and now, against all odds and professional expectations, he is back at work.

The human body and mind are capable of the most amazing feats of recovery and regeneration. Vicky, who had had not one but two of Clare's operations, was a prize example, and we heard of another from our friend Jenni who visited Clare on Maundy Thursday. Jenni is the former nurse who now runs the retirement home in the New Forest. She came clumping in with a broken ankle in plaster but radiating all her usual cheerfulness and confidence and carrying a gorgeous white polar bear. He had a silver bell round his neck and silver sparkles in his shining fur. 'Oh, he's lovely!' exclaimed Clare, as she hugged this latest addition to the already extensive menagerie of fluffy animals which shared her bed. At the same time I could see that Jenni was casting a professional eye over her and was relieved by what she saw. Then she told us of the last time she had visited the London Hospital, about five years ago, when she visited the twenty-year old daughter of some great friends. This young woman had been in a coma for over four months after a car accident, then one morning, as a nurse bent over her to lift her eyelids and shine a torch in them, she suddenly opened her eyes of her own accord, reached out her hand to take a ball-point pen from the nurse's pocket, and proceeded to sign her name dozens and dozens of times all over the sheets. It was the start of another miraculous recovery. She is now

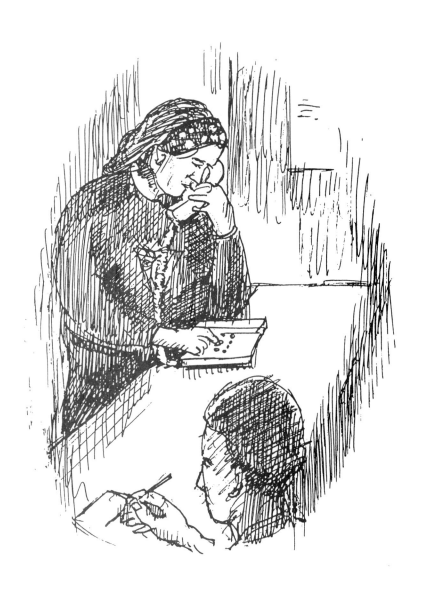

happily married and with a family of her own.

Of course there are failures too, and by the very nature of a Trauma Unit designed to look after the victims of the most serious accidents, it has a lot of disappointments and sadnesses. When I told Jenni how wonderful the staff there were and how they kept coming across to see Clare on their way home, she explained to me that they needed the encouragement of seeing success. To see Vicky going home to play her cello again and, God willing, Clare following a similar path of recovery, was a tremendous boost to their morale. I had not thought of it in those terms, but then I remembered Dr Britto's remark when Clare had been trying to use the telephone at the front desk the other evening: 'This is what makes it all worthwhile'.

The staff in Garden House were a good team too. If less high-powered than the Trauma Unit nurses, they were highly competent in their less technological type of care and they were all very kind. There was a good atmosphere everywhere, and even the humblest domestic staff were concerned and caring. There was one man in particular who did the floors every day with a special machine which applied a non-slippery polish and kept down the dust. His English was rather limited, but he always asked after the patients and was so careful not to bang the beds of children who were in them. It sounds only a little thing, but as a veteran of a lot of painful spinal carpentry myself many years ago I still wince at the recollection of clumsy cleaners who would jolt the bed and were impervious to requests to be a little more careful. As for the nursing staff, they were such a good team that it would be invidious to pick anyone out for special mention except for 'Pavarotti', who was so unusual that he must qualify as an exception to any rule.

His real name was Keith, and he was the only male nurse in Garden House. I called him Pavarotti because he was built on the same generous scale as the great singer, and when I first saw him he was going home wearing a Pavarotti-style cardigan with a tremendous roll-collar. He was a giant of a man, nearly six feet tall and weighing at least eighteen stones, but as gentle as a kitten. He was enormous fun and always on the look-out for things to do to cheer the children up. When he asked Clare what London shows she had seen, she could not remember without prompting, but when he whistled some of the tunes she recognised them at once - particularly the Lambeth Walk and other songs from 'Me and My Girl', which she had greatly enjoyed. It turned out to be one of Keith's favourites too - he was a great show-goer - and the next day he popped in with a tape of that musical and some light classical music on the other side. Of course, once you get tunes like that into your head you can't get them out again, and for days afterwards I was forever 'Doing the Lambeth Walk' or observing that 'The sun has got his hat on and he's coming out today'.

Clare was rather overwhelmed with visitors on Good Friday, particularly after the excitement of the navy's visit, but though she got very tired she kept having little naps and perking up again. The Bulmers came and were thrilled to see her progress. Doreen came too, and so did some of Clare's school friends. I could tell she was getting better when I saw her sitting cross-legged on the bed chattering away to the voluble Charlie and Alice, and though she often got the words wrong, it did not seem to matter. It was more important that she was getting over the shyness about making mistakes. As with learning a foreign language - or trying to speak a once well-known but long unused one - it is important to 'have a go' and not worry too much about getting it perfect first time. Anyway Alice and Charlie did not seem put off, and as they all seemed to be talking at once, as teenage girls do, they may not even have noticed.

About tea-time we had a lovely surprise. Ros came in with Mr Sutcliffe, Clare's surgeon. Ros wanted to be sure that we had all we needed to carry on Clare's exercise programme over the long week-end, and Mr Sutcliffe, having examined Clare, said, 'Well, young lady, it's about time you saw your own home. You can go home for the day tomorrow if you like, though I shall want you back in the evening'. What a wonderful Easter gift! Easter Saturday would be exactly two weeks from the day of her accident. When I had a word with Mr Sutcliffe in the corridor, even that most cautious of men could not conceal his delight at Clare's progress and her lack of any of the common psychological problems he had warned us to expect.

'May I shake your hand again now?' I asked, remembering how worried he had been that I should not expect too much for Clare when I had asked to shake his hand before, when she had just come off the ventilator and her life seemed out of danger.

'Yes', he said, 'with pleasure. There is still a long way to go and I can't guarantee a complete recovery, but I am very pleased with her progress. She's right at the top end of our spectrum of expectations.

She's been a very lucky girl.'

'She has been very lucky to be in this hospital and have you for her surgeon', I said, and I have never shaken a man's hand with greater sincerity or sense of obligation.

CHAPTER TWELVE

The blackbird in the little courtyard outside Garden House woke me up about half past four on Easter Saturday morning. It was a beautiful dawn, the air was like champagne, and it promised to be a glorious day. It would have been a glorious day for us of course if it had been pouring with rain, but nature was in perfect harmony with our mood this morning. The only worry we had was that Clare seemed to have a slight infection of the waterworks and intimate regions, but antibiotics were reducing her frequencies and Mary had been given cream to apply too. Mary was in fact advancing on Clare with the cream when I turned up to see them about seven o'clock, for as I was about to open the door I heard an indignant 'That's more than enough!' from the recipient.

After breakfast and a bath we got the final go-ahead to take Clare home. I went to fetch the car and told Mary that I should be at the back entrance, but in the excitement Mary had misheard and wheeled Clare to the front instead. Never mind, we got our act together eventually, and were far too happy to be grumpy with each other. We were glad we had an estate car as it was so easy to put the wheel-chair in the back. We sat Clare in the back seat without a problem - taking great care not to let her bang her head - and Mary sat next to her while I chauffeured. We were home in twenty-five minutes, and when we arrived, Clare was able to walk into the house with a little help and did not need the chair.

The first thing she wanted was the toilet, which meant going upstairs, but she managed it without difficulty and came down safely holding the banister rail while I went in front and Mary came behind in case she slipped. Then we installed her on the sofa in the sitting room and opened the French windows to let the beautiful spring air in, full of the scents of hyacinths, late narcissi and jasmine. I brought the wheel-chair in, and when she was rested I pushed her out into the garden while Mary prepared a lunch of all her favourite easily-digestibles - roast chicken with all the trimmings, trifle and some sparkling apple juice which looked like champagne.

Far from being sleepy after lunch, Clare was full of life. Whereas adults tend to become torpid, a child's response to serious refuelling is often an immediate desire to expend energy, so we started her exercises on the lawn. Then we did a little quiz. First I asked her to match a list of authors to a list of her favourite books, but though she scored higher than the previous day, she was still quite hazy. Mathematically, however, she was on very good form and wrote in the correct amounts for the following questions almost as soon as she had read them.

'Today is 18th April and it is Saturday. What date will next Saturday be?'

'I am fourteen and this is 1992. In what year will I be twenty?'

'Jim bought 4 pears at 5p each. How much change did he get from 50p?'

'Mary bought 2 bars of chocolate at 10p each and 4 yoghurts at 20p each. How much did it all cost?'

'Daddy is driving at 30 m.p.h. How long will it take him to go 60 miles?'

It is a long way from differential calculus, admittedly, but only a week ago we were still wondering if Clare would even be able to talk. Then finally I copied out some simple sentences from the first lesson in her Italian course-book, and though she seemed to have lost her active vocabulary she understood the sentences immediately.

Joanna and Frances both came to see her in the afternoon, then she had a little sleep until tea-time when our elderly next-door neighbours, who were looking after her budgerigar, came in. She perked up at once and joined in the conversation, not always finding the right words but generally comprehensible. Not surprisingly after all the excitement as well as the exertions of the day she was getting tired, and when we took her back to the hospital about 6 o'clock she went straight to bed - only to be roused half an hour later by the supper trolley, to which she did full justice despite the huge lunch she had eaten at home! Then she became highly talkative and was on terrific form when Steve from the Trauma Unit popped in to see her on his way home and talked to her about the helicopter. Steve was delighted with her progress. She now understood who he was and, in a vague way, what had happened, though she could not remember being in the Trauma Unit at all. We all slept very well that night.

When I came down to Clare's room at 7.15 the next morning, Easter Sunday, I found her already up and about to have a bath. She had breakfast sitting in an ordinary chair, then at 8.15 we sat her in the wheel-chair and pushed her across to the Chapel for the

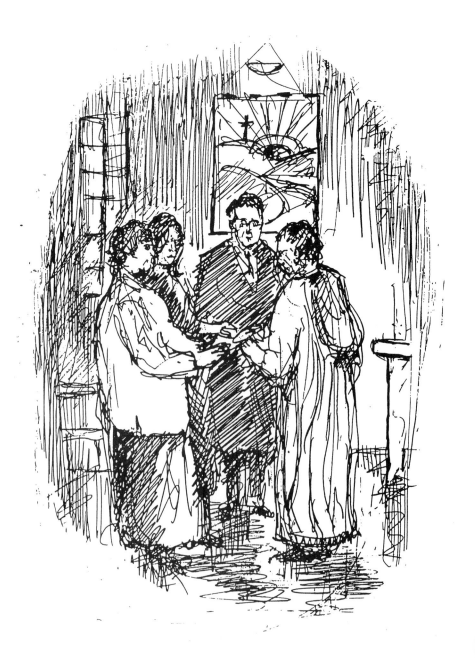

Communion service at 8.30. Our friend the Chaplain was there, together with his two assistants, and there was a small congregation of patients and relatives. The little Chapel looked lovely. The sun was streaming through the stained-glass windows representing the Resurrection, and the tall Easter candles were ready to be lit. Clare insisted on walking in and sitting in an ordinary chair.

The service began with the hymn 'Jesus Christ is risen today', which the Chaplain himself accompanied on the piano, and Clare sang the words from the hymn-book without hesitation. She also followed all the responses in the service-book, and when the moment of Communion came, she had no trouble in standing to receive the bread and wine. It was deeply moving. In the prayers that followed the Chaplain said we should all thank God for personal aspects of the Resurrection which we had experienced in life, and we knew exactly what he meant.

After the service we went up in the lift to the Trauma Unit where we found Sandra and Sarah-Jane on duty. We left the wheel-chair outside and Clare walked in to receive the biggest hugs she had ever had. We were all so happy, and just as we felt it was impossible to be happier, we saw Carole Davies in the corridor and heard good news about Len. He was responding at last to the treatment, his kidneys were starting to work again, and Carole was once again full of hope, which this time would not prove false. Then to cap it all, as soon as we got Clare back to Garden House, 'Pavarotti' brought in Jack, the little baby who had been so ill in an oxygen tent when Clare had first come into the paediatric unit. The tiny little thing was now fully recovered, gurgling happily in the cradle of Keith's enormous hands, and when Keith let Clare hold him for a moment I have never seen a happier smile. How very different from that distant, expressionless icon-like face Clare had had when she first came into Garden House. It was a wonderful Easter.

From that day on Clare never looked back. The following Friday she went home for good, and though there were three months of rehabilitation to come, with regular visits to the physio gym as an outpatient, physical and mental exercise programmes at home, two hours a week at a Tutorial College on Maths and English, Italian lessons at home and constant attention from Mary and me, who had to make big changes in our working lives to ensure that one or other of us could be with her the whole time, it was worth every minute when

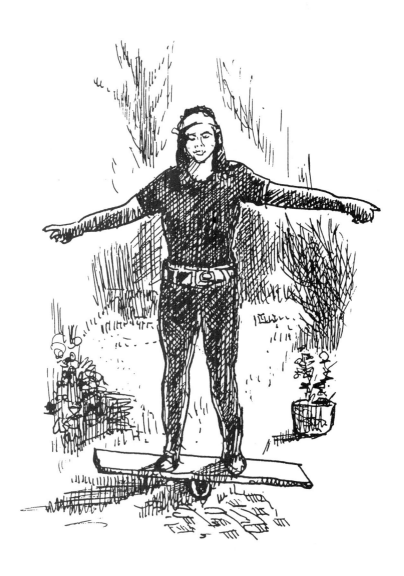

she went back to school for the start of the Michaelmas term in September as though nothing had happened since she was last there. Her hair had grown again to cover the scars, and apart from being forbidden 'rough' games like hockey that could give her a bang on the head, she was able to participate fully in school life, cope with all the lessons and resume all her friendships and activities. We celebrated her return to school with another visit to the hospital Chapel, and as we came out we saw one of the nurses from Garden House who asked anxiously, 'What are *you* doing here? There's nothing wrong is there?' 'Nothing at all', I replied. 'We've just been to the service in the Chapel. We've such a lot to be thankful for'. But how can anyone express what it feels like to have witnessed a miracle, a modern miracle of healing that is no less wonderful because it depended on the God-given skills of surgeons and nurses reinforced by the love and prayers of so many dear friends and loved ones?

EPILOGUE

If this had been a novel I could have done what Victorian authors did and told my readers what happened to the characters afterwards, which could be a future of undiluted bliss. As it is, I can predict nothing because my characters are real people, and Heaven only knows what the rest of their lives have in store for them. My happy ending is the simple fact that it is the beginning of the rest of their lives for Clare, Len Davies, Vicky and all the other patients who have not just been kept in existence but have been restored to mental and physical health through the skill and dedication of the story's heroes and heroines - the surgical, medical, nursing, physiotherapy and support staff of the Royal London Hospital's specialist Trauma Unit which works these modern miracles of healing.

What I can do, however, is to say what I should like to see happen in the future. I should like to see the work of this unit better known and appreciated. That indeed is one of the main reasons why I wrote this book. I wanted to give life and personal meaning to the bare statistics which I mentioned in my *Preface* and repeat here. The usual expectation in any series of patients of the type treated by the London's Trauma Unit would be for 15 per cent to be left in a permanent vegetative state and for a further fifteen to twenty per cent to be so severely incapacitated as to be unable to live independent lives. The reality is that there have been no such outcomes in either category since this experimental unit began. Anecdotally there have also been patients who according to all the textbooks should not have survived but are fully restored, physically and mentally.

Now let us put some numbers to this astonishing record, numbers of real people like Clare, Vicky or Len. According to *Headway,* the National Head Injuries Association, of the one million people who attend hospitals in this country each year as a result of head injury, 'about 10,000 will suffer moderate brain-damage causing unconsciousness for up to six hours: some of these will have physical and cognitive defects after five years and a few will not work again. A further 4,500 will suffer severe brain-injuries involving unconsciousness for six hours or longer: of these only 15 per cent will have returned to work within five years, and many will not work again'. Moreover, even among the less impaired, there is often the danger of post-traumatic epilepsy with all its attendant problems for a return to work, such as inability to drive a car or to do any job involving climbing ladders or scaffolding. Now the figures I have just given are annual ones, and because so many of the victims of severe brain injury are young people and their life expectancies long, the total number of survivors of the latter category alone - the severely brain-injured - is estimated by *Headway* at 'almost 100,000'. This means that if all future victims of severe head-injury were to have access to a specialist Trauma Service like that pioneered at the London, there would be the potential to restore to the population of the country up to 30,000 useful and independent lives.

Not surprisingly, therefore, when I took Mary and Clare to see our friends at the Trauma Unit to wish them a Merry (1993) Christmas, we were dismayed to find them apprehensive about the future because the unit was still 'experimental' and 'being evaluated'. Naturally it is not cheap to operate, though it is run on a shoe-string compared with equivalents in America. But its results are unsurpassed anywhere in the world. The savings in terms of human suffering, both of patients and their families, are of course incalculable, but even in the most rigorous of purely financial cost-benefit analyses the tangible costs of operating the Unit must be compared not only with savings of public money which would otherwise have been needed to support the highly dependent patients but also with the loss of earning capacity of the patients and their carers and with the many other financial implications of shattered lives, families and careers.

Headway knows this better than anyone because it picks up the pieces. 'Brain-injury', it writes, 'occurs most commonly in males between the ages of 17 and 27. Forty per cent are the result of road traffic accidents, and 16 per cent will have some additional injury. Even in cases of a severe disablement, life-span may not be shortened. The period of dependence and need is therefore extended over many years. In such circumstances the burden of care places the family unit under great strain. The financial liabilities upon those in support, including the appropriate Department of State, are extensive. These aspects are lessened in each case where the outcome of head injury can be improved'. But when *Headway* and other charities begin their wonderful work of support and rehabilitation, the damage has been done. This is why, if I could write the policy of the Department of Health over the next few years, I should plan to provide national coverage by cloning the London's Trauma Unit, including the Helicopter Emergency Medical Service, in a sufficient number of major regional hospitals with strong neurosurgical departments.

A second purpose for writing this book which I should like to see fulfilled is the raising of money for charity, for author's royalties of ten per cent of the sale price will go to the Neurosurgical Fund of the London Hospital and to other related medical and rehabilitation charities, and the entire net proceeds of books sold through a charity will of course go to that charity. A third aim was to bring some light among the prevailing gloom and, increasingly, sheer nastiness of so much that is written today or considered newsworthy. We hear so much about young people going wrong but so little about the quiet dedication, decency, humanity and skill of the young miracle-workers whom I was privileged to meet and get to know.

Finally I thought that this story might help other families who find themselves confronting a similar disaster, and the friends of such families. At the same time I am very conscious of how lucky we were with Clare, for while the speed and completeness of her recovery are far from unique - and will become more common if specialist Trauma Units become available to more accident-victims - there will be many healings that take a lot longer and others that are never so complete. There will also be cases of severe dependency, and God knows my heart goes out to them and their families. From our own mercifully brief experience, however, and from what I have subsequently discovered, perhaps I could offer a few words of advice.

In the sudden shock of the accident and the days that follow, do not despair. However horrific the patient looks, remember that a severely head-injured child who was deeply unconscious, going cold and needing open-brain surgery to save her life, was conscious again and beginning to recover her faculties in less than two weeks. But remember too that coma can continue for much longer without necessarily involving permanent impairment. Remember our friend Jenni's story of visiting a brain-injured young woman who was in a coma for nearly six months and is now married with a family of her own. Admittedly that is at the other end of the time-spectrum from Clare, but again it is not unique. My neurologist friend Professor Hughie Webb told me of a similar case when he was a young hospital doctor doing a locum at a hospital in Exeter many years ago, long before the development of the techniques that made Clare's miracle possible. He had wondered if it was worthwhile keeping alive a medical student who had been struck by a car on the Exeter by-pass and had been in a deep coma for many months, devoid of reflexes or movement. When he went to do the same locum a year later my friend found the young man still there in the hospital, but this time wearing a white coat and accompanying his fellow medical students on the ward-rounds.

To relatives and friends of a patient's immediate family I should recommend writing lots of little cards and messages or ringing regularly to let them know that you are thinking about them, but when it comes to visiting think carefully first. The immediate family will be in a state of shock, may want to be alone with the patient and may not want others to see how terrible the patient looks. If you do visit, keep it short, and do not insist on seeing the patient if you sense that the immediate family may not wish it or if you feel you may break down. It may be better to take the patient's parents or children for a cup of tea either in the hospital canteen or, more privately, in the room that is normally reserved for the relatives of patients in Trauma or Intensive Therapy units. It is the immediate family rather than the patient that you are helping at this stage. Be careful too what you say. Don't say for instance 'I know how you must feel' unless you really do, which could only be because you have experienced the same thing yourself. Let the person you are visiting say what he or she wants, and if they break down and weep it is probably the best thing to relieve them. Above all, be ready to offer practical help to reduce their other worries. Whether it is looking after a dependent child or granny or just a family pet, contacting an employer or school to explain matters, helping to deal with a financial or legal problem, helping to arrange disability aids and equipment for the return home or just offering lifts in your car, try to discover needs and anticipate requests.

Most hospital's social workers, rehabilitation experts and other support services will be very helpful in preparing for the patient's return home, but do remember there are many other sources of help, and relatives and friends can perform a great service by contacting some of these, finding out about local support groups and organising aids and special equipment that may be needed. I have given brief details of some of them. Remember too that the family will need more, not less, support when the patient has returned to consciousness and begins the often long process of rehabilitation, beginning in hospital and continuing at home. We were very lucky with Clare, but many brain-injured patients suffer profound psychological and personality changes, the most common of which are extreme irritability and lack of social inhibitions both in language and behaviour. Usually this is a passing phase but it can often be a matter of many months rather than weeks, and highly stressful while it lasts. Relatives and friends who rushed around helping when the accident first happened now begin to find many easy excuses for keeping away, but just imagine what the immediate family is going through. Rehabilitation, even where recovery is ultimately complete, takes time, patience and understanding.

The importance of *continuing* support is nowhere better emphasised than in a little book which, unlike mine, does not have a happy ending. This is *Karen's Diary,* published by *Headway* and available from the address given under *Sources of Information, Advice and Help* on page 139. It is a young wife's record of her feelings and experiences after her husband suffered severe head-injuries in a motorbike accident. Karen and Malcolm were a happily married young couple with two children, a toddler of two years and a baby of four months. Karen's account shows how nursing and treatment appear to someone who is in a state of shock and helplessness, how individual members of staff and family and friends reacted to the distress, anger, confusion and practical problems of a young wife whose husband has been suddenly transformed from a supportive and loving father to a very different and dependent stranger. Gradually her old circle of friends forsook her, the tensions increased, and when she finally admitted failure in an increasingly lonely struggle she was cruelly criticised by relatives and friends who had passed by on the other side when she had most needed their help. It is a starkly honest and moving account which those involved in evaluating the work of the London's Trauma Unit could usefully read alongside this book - not because of any necessary relevance to the particular cases in these two accounts but because they exemplify the very different kind of life that a specialist Trauma Unit can provide for some 30 per cent of severely brain-injured accident-victims (and their families) who would otherwise end up in a state of high dependence for the rest of their lives.

SOURCES OF INFORMATION, ADVICE AND HELP

Reference books and useful publications

One of the best reference books is the *Directory for Disabled People,* compiled by Ann Darnbrough and Derek Kinrade and published by Woodhead-Faulkner in association with the **Royal Association for Disability and Rehabilitation (RADAR).** This comprehensive and regularly updated handbook is available in many book shops and most public libraries and Citizens' Advice Bureaux. It has sections on the Statutory Services (which are legally required to be provided by the State and Local Authorities), Benefits and Allowances, Aids and Equipment, House and Home, Education, Mobility and Motoring, Holidays, Sex and Personal Relations, Contact Organisations, Helpful Organisations and where to find advice on such specialist areas as compensation claims for personal injury or medical negligence. It sounds formidable, but it is in fact easy to use, being carefully compiled, clearly written and well cross-referenced.

Many of the specialist charities also produce some very useful publications, often short booklets by experts on specific matters such as activities for the head-injured person at home, education after head-injury, understanding and dealing with emotional and behavioural problems, getting back to school or work, helping children cope with a parent's head-injury and general guidelines for helpers over the rehabilitation period. As a start I should advise contacting at least **Headway** and **MENCAP** for their lists of publications, also where appropriate the **Children's Head Injury Trust.** Their addresses are given on pages 133-4. **RADAR** itself also has many excellent publications: its address is 25 Mortimer Street, London, W1N 8AB (telephone 071 637 5400).

Citizens' Advice Bureaux

Local **Citizens' Advice Bureaux** provide information and advice on every subject, free of charge. There are over a thousand of them spread throughout the country, and you will find the address and telephone number of your nearest one in the telephone directory or by asking at your local library. While they differ in size and depth of expertise, all of them have a community information system including addresses of self-help groups, local charities and indeed local solicitors who specialise in compensation claims. Some have specialist debt counsellors on the staff, but all Bureau workers are trained to deal with money problems. They will also make telephone calls and appointments and write letters for anyone who cannot cope.

Advice on disability generally

DIAL UK (National Association of Disablement Information and Advice Lines) are autonomous local associations of people with personal experience of disability and with the primary aim of providing information to other disabled people or those involved in helping them. A telephone call or letter to the head office will give you details of the local association. The head office address is Park Lodge, St Catherine's Hospital, Tickhill Road, Balby, Doncaster, DN4 8QN (telephone 0302 310123).

There are also some regionally based information services. The **Northern Ireland Council on Disability (NICD)** at 2 Annadale Avenue, Belfast, BT7 3JR (telephone 0232 491011) is an independent voluntary organisation representing every aspect of disability with over 130 member organisations. Its information office is open from 10 a.m. to 4 p.m. Monday to Friday. Wales has the **Wales Council for the Disabled (Cyngor Cymru I'r Anabl),** which can be contacted at 'Llys Ifor', Crescent Road, Caerphilly, CF8 1XL (telephone 0222 887325). In Scotland, in addition to the 64 Citizens' Advice Bureaux and 25 affiliated agencies supported by **Citizens' Advice Scotland,** there is **Disability Scotland** at 5 Shandwick Place, Edinburgh, EH2 4RG (telephone 031 229 8632) and **Wellbeing,** a Glasgow-based information service specialising in the formation of self-help groups to enable people with similar problems to make contact with each other: its address is Volunteer Centre, 25-27 Elmbank Street, Glasgow, G2 4PB (telephone 041 226 3431).

For advice on technical aids, equipment and services for disabled people the **Disabled Living Foundation** provides a comprehensive information service from its head office at 380-384 Harrow Road, London, W9 2HU (telephone 071 289 6111), which also has a permanent collection of aids and equipment on display. Its information service is open from 9.30 a.m. to 4.45 p.m. Monday to Friday, and a useful selection of publications is available to the disabled free of charge. The same offices also house the headquarters of the **DLCC,** The Disabled Living Centres Council (telephone 071 266 2059), which is the representative body for a large number of regional centres throughout Great Britain: a call to the head office will give you details of the nearest centre to your home. *There is also an excellent section on Aids and Equipment, with many useful contact addresses, in the Directory for Disabled People.*

Advice and help specifically for the brain-injured

Headway (National Head Injuries Association), set up in 1979, now has nearly a hundred local groups in Britain and 23 Rehabilitation Day Centres. It provides advice and counselling centres in many towns and cities, regional rehabilitation and care training centres, and respite homes to give short-term relief to long-term carers. Through its local groups it gives advice and support to the head-injured and their families, help in the rehabilitation programmes of patients in the home, social and leisure activities and opportunities for those involved to meet others and share experiences. Families faced with having to cope with a brain-injury and rehabilitation should not hesitate to contact Headway at 7 King Edward Court, King Edward Street, Nottingham, NG1 1EW (telephone 0602 240800).

The Children's Head Injury Trust was set up to find out more about the effects of head injury in children, to pass onto parents information on the care of these children and to support parents who feel they do not know where to turn. The Trust provides some excellent information sheets specially written for parents to give them some basic information in the early days following their child's injury, including the mechanisms of a head injury, who's who in the hospital, a general account of physical disabilities, a list of useful agencies and some preliminary notes on rehabilitation. A further set of leaflets covers rehabilitation in more detail, what to look for, fits, rehabilitation of physical difficulties, communication, problems in thinking and learning, emotional and behavioural problems, friends and friendships, the effect on brothers and sisters, returning to school, the 'statementing process' (which is the process by which special educational needs are assessed and met) and practical guidance for children with a legal claim for compensation for their injuries. These leaflets and further information about the Trust and its Family Support Groups should be obtained by parents or a relative or friend of the stricken family as soon as possible after the accident from Children's Head Injury Trust, c/o Neurosurgery, The Radcliffe Infirmary, Woodstock Road, Oxford, OX2 6HE (telephone 0865 224786), or through Headway.

MENCAP (The Royal Society for Mentally Handicapped Children and Adults) is the largest organisation for people with a learning disability, their parents and families. Learning disability is defined as a permanent condition caused by impairment or injury of the brain, which can have a wide variety of causes including genetic defects, maternal infections during pregnancy, childhood infections such as encephalitis or meningitis, injury to the baby during labour or birth or head injuries caused by assault or road accidents. Mencap provides support for families and individuals through its 500 local Mencap groups, housing in the community for some 2,400 people with learning disabilities, employment and training through its Pathway Employment Service and training colleges, short-term respite care holidays, leisure opportunities in the community through its 700 Gateway clubs and leisure projects and further education through its three colleges of further education. Its head office is The Mencap Centre at 123 Golden Lane, London, EC1Y 0RT (telephone 071 454 0454) and it has seven divisional offices covering England, Wales and Northern Ireland. The London Division and Southern Division both operate from the head office and use the same telephone number. The other five are Northern Division at Harrogate (0423 568162), Western Division at Birmingham (021 356 7306), Eastern Division at Stamford (0780 51199), Mencap in Wales at Cardiff (0222 494933) and Mencap in Northern Ireland at Belfast (0232 691351). In Scotland the equivalent but quite separate charity is the **Scottish Society for the Mentally Handicapped,** which operates through 70 branches providing a variety of services for the mentally handicapped and their families. Its head office is at 13 Elmbank Street, Glasgow, G2 4QA (telephone 041 226 4541).

Advice and help for the spine-injured

This book is mainly about head injuries, but sometimes spinal cord injuries are involved too, with the prospect of a permanent degree of paralysis. The principal charity providing help and advice in this area is the **Spinal Injuries Association (SIA).** Run with superb efficiency by paraplegics and tetraplegics, the SIA has an Information Service to answer any queries, a Welfare Service to help with problems and confidential matters, a Personal Assistance Service to provide assistance when it is needed most, a Personal Injury Claims Service, a number of helpful publications and some holiday accommodation including a specially adapted narrowboat. Its national headquarters is at 76 St James's Lane, London N1O 3DF (telephone 081 444 2121). There is also a completely confidential crisis counselling line, which is 081 883 4296.